VIVAs In Surgical Anatomy

James Crichton BSc MBChB MRCS

Andrew Davies BSc MBChB MRCS PGCert. (Clinical ed.)

Mothana Gawad BSc MBBS MRCS PGCert. (Clinical ed.)

© 2016 MD+ Publishing

www.mdbookpublishing.com

Published by: MD+ Publishing

Cover Design: Alexander Logan

ISBN-10: 0993113885

ISBN-13: 978-0-993113888

Printed in the United Kingdom

Acknowledgements

The authors would like to thank the following staff at King's College London for their guidance and support during the production of this text:

Dr Andrew Hunter and Miss Barbara Webb for facilitating the project in the Anatomy Department at King's.

Dr Mike Hutchinson and Mr David Parry for permission to photograph their excellent prosections.

The dissection room manager Kirsty and support staff Stella, Doug and Holly for kindly sourcing the specimens.

Professor Harold Ellis for his unrivalled teaching and for reviewing earlier drafts of the manuscript.

CONTENTS

3: Thorax

4: Lower Limb

5: Upper Limb

6: Spine

Foreword - Professor Harold Ellis

I am delighted to have been asked by the authors of this excellent volume to provide its Foreword. No one could possibly argue with me that a sound knowledge of Anatomy is the basis of clinical examination of the patient, of safe operative surgery and of the interpretation of radiological images and now of the increasingly sophisticated images obtained by ultrasound, computerized tomography and nuclear magnetic resonance.

To obtain this knowledge, nothing can surpass the dissection and study of the cadaver, but this is becoming more and more difficult in this country as something like one in three of the medical schools in the United Kingdom have lost, (or never possessed), an Anatomy department. A helpful aid to learning and revision for examination candidates is provided by this excellent atlas of dissections, osteological specimens and radiological images, with their accompanying questions and answers.

To those of you preparing for the Anatomy component of your examinations, especially the MRCS, I recommend a careful study of the images and text contained in this volume.

Professor Harold Ellis CBE FRCS

Glossary of Anatomical Eponyms

Eponymous terms are frequently encountered in the MRCS examination. They are presented alphabetically below.

Baker's Cyst
A bulging of the synovial cavity of the knee posteriorly into the popliteal space. Often associated with knee arthritis. William Morrant Baker (1838-1896), Surgeon at St Bartholomew's Hospital, London, UK.

Barrett's Oesophagus
Intestinal metaplasia of the cells lining the lower oesophagus, from normal stratified squamous epithelium to simple columnar. Significantly associated with oesophageal cancer. Norman Barrett (1903-1979), Consultant Thoracic Surgeon to St. Thomas' Hospital, London, UK.

Venous Plexus of Batson
A venous network connecting the deep pelvic and thoracic veins, forming a route for metastatic pelvic cancer spread, typically from the rectum or prostate, to the spine. Oscar Vivian Batson (1894-1979), Anatomist.

Beck's Triad
Signs associated with acute cardiac tamponade – hypotension, muffled heart sounds and jugular venous distension. The complete triad is rarely seen in tamponade, but if all are present it is pathognomonic. Claude Beck (1894-1971), Professor of Cardiac Surgery, Case Western Reserve University, Pennsylvania, USA.

Bennett's Fracture
Intra-articular fracture of the base of the first metacarpal. Edward Hallaran Bennett (1937-1907), Professor of Surgery, Trinity College Dublin.

Bouchard's Nodes
Bony outgrowths found at the proximal interphalangeal joints in osteoarthritis and rheumatoid arthritis (cf. Heberden's nodes). Charles Bouchard (1837-1915), Chair of Pathology at Bicetre Hospital, France.

Broca's Area
A region in the dominant frontal lobe linked to speech production. Pierre Paul Broca (1824-1880), Professor of Clinical Surgery at the Academie de Medicine, Paris, France.

Buck's Fascia
The deep fascia of the penis, continuous with the external spermatic fascia. Gurdon Buck (1807-1877), Plastic Surgeon, New York, USA.

Bundle of His
Part of the conducting pathway of the heart – specialised cardiac muscle

cells that conduct the impulse from the atrioventricular node to the fascicular branches. Wihelm His Jr. (1863-1934), Professor of Medicine at the University of Berlin, Germany.

Calot's Triangle
Also known as the hepatobilary triangle, this is a space bordered by the common hepatic duct, cystic duct and the inferior border of the liver. Important in gallbladder surgery, as the cystic artery is found here. Jean-Francois Calot (1861-1944), French Surgeon.

Cloquet's Node
The single lymph node found in the femoral canal. Jules Germain Cloquet (1790-1883), Physician and Surgeon, Paris, France.

Colles' Fracture
Extra-articular fracture of the distal radius with dorsal displacement of the wrist and hand. Typically caused by a fall onto the outstretched hand. Abraham Colles (1773-1843), Professor of Anatomy, Surgery and Physiology at the Royal College of Surgeons in Ireland.

Colles' Fascia
The deep layer of the superficial perineal fascia.

Suspensory Ligaments of Cooper
Found in the breast, running from the clavicle and clavipectoral fascia to the breast parenchyma, suspending the breast and giving it its shape. Sir Astley Paston Cooper (1768-1841), Surgeon and Anatomist at Guy's Hospital, London, UK.

Cushing's Response
Or Cushing's reflex, this describes hypertension, bradycardia and irregular breathing seen with drastically raised intracranial pressure. Harvey Cushing (1869-1939), Sterling Professor of Neurology at Yale University, USA and "the father of modern Neurosurgery".

DeBakey Classification
Another classification system for aortic dissection. DeBakey I involves the ascending aorta and propagates to the descending. DeBakey II is limited to the ascending aorta only and DeBakey III is in limited to the descending. Michael E DeBakey (1908 – 2008), Cardiac Surgeon and Chancellor Emeritus at Baylor College of Medicine, Houston, Texas, USA.

Down Syndrome
Genetic disorder caused by trisomy of chromosome 21, producing characteristic physical defects, variable cognitive deficit and cardiac problems. John Langdon Down (1828 – 1896), physician at the London Hospital, England.

Marginal Artery of Drummond
A large blood vessel that travels in the colonic mesentery and forms an anastomosis between the superior and inferior mesenteric arteries. Sir David Drummond (1852-1932), Physician and Professor of the Principles and Practice of Medicine, University of Durham, UK.

Dukes' Staging
A staging system for colorectal cancer, staging the disease from A to D. Cuthbert Dukes (1890-1977), Pathologist at St. Mark's Hospital, London, UK.

Erb-Duchenne Paralysis
A paralysis affecting the upper nerve roots of the brachial plexus, most commonly affecting the suprascapular, musculocutaneous and axillary nerve. Guillaume Benjamin Amand Duchenne (1806-1875), French neurologist and Wilhelm Heinrich Erb (1840-1921), German neurologist.

Fallot's Tetralogy
Congenital heart defect characterized by; pulmonary stenosis, right ventricular hypertrophy, ventricular septal defect and an overriding aorta. Etienne-Louis Arthur Fallot (1850-1911), French Physician.

Finkelstein's Test
A test of tenosynovitis of the abductor pollicis longus and extensor pollicis longus tendons, performed by grasping the thumb and pulling it and the wrist into ulnar deviation. Harry Finkelstein (1855-1939), American surgeon.

Frey's syndrome
A syndrome resulting from damage to the auriculotemporal branch of the trigeminal nerve. This carries parasympathetic fibres to the parotid gland and sweat glands of the face and scalp. Faulty regeneration of these nerve fibres may result in gustatory sweating, where sweating occurs instead of the normal salivatory response. Lucja Frey (1889-1942), Polish Physician and Neurologist.

Galeazzi Fracture
A fracture of the distal radius with dislocation of the distal radioulnar joint. Ricardo Galeazzi (1866-1952) Professor of Orthopaedic Surgery, Milan.

Garden Classification
Four stage classification of intracapsular neck of femur fractures. Robert Symon Garden (1910-1982), orthopaedic surgeon to the Preston and Chorley Group of Hospitals.

Guyon's Canal
Longitudinal canal of the wrist that transmits the ulnar artery and ulnar nerve. Jean Casimir Felix Guyon (1831-1920) Professor of surgical pathology and later Professor of genitourinary surgery, University of Paris.

Heinz Bodies
Small round inclusions within red blood cells formed from denatured haemoglobin, seen in haemolytic anaemia, inborn errors of metabolism, alpha-thalassaemia and chronic liver disease. Robert Heinz (1865-1924), German Physician.

Hesselbach's triangle
Part of the anterior abdominal wall through which direct inguinal hernia occur. Bordered by lateral border of the rectus sheath, the inferior epigastric artery and the inguinal ligament. Franz Kaspar Hesselbach (1759-1816), German Surgeon and Anatomist.

Horner's Syndrome
A syndrome resulting from damage to the sympathetic trunk, innervating the eyelids and pupil. Characterised by miosis, ptosis and anhidrosis. Johann Friedrich Horner (1831-1886), Swiss Ophthalmologist.

Howell-Jolly Bodies
Basophilic nuclear remnants seen in red blood cells, seen with decreased splenic function or post-splenectomy. William Henry Howell (1860-1945), American Physiologist and Justin Marie Jolly (1870-1953), French Haematologist.

Hunter's Canal
A canal located the medial thigh and extending from the apex of the femoral triangle to the adductor hiatus. John Hunter (1728-1793), surgeon at St George's Hospital, London.

Killian's Dehiscence
Pharyngoesophageal diverticulum found in the inferior constrictor of the pharaynx between the thyropharyngeus and cricopharyngeus muscles. Gustav Killian (1820-1889), German Laryngologist.

Lachman's Test
A test of the integrity of the anterior cruciate ligament, performed with the knee flexed to 20 degrees. The tibia is translated anteriorly on the femoral condyles by the examiner. Considered superior to the anterior drawer test. John Lachman, Chairman of Orthopaedic Surgery and Sports Medicine, Philadelphia, USA.

Lisfranc Fracture
A fracture of one or more metatarsals, with displacement of the metatarsal bones from the tarsus. Jacques Lisfranc de St. Martin (1790-1847), French Surgeon and Gynaecologist at the time of the Napoleonic wars.

Dorsal Tubercle of Lister
Bony prominence found on the dorsal surface of the distal radius. Joseph Lister (1827-1912), Professor of Surgery at the University of Glasgow, and subsequently the University of Edinburgh and King's College London.

Long Thoracic Nerve of Bell
Nerve supplying the serratus anterior muscle, most commonly arising from C5-C7. Sir Charles Bell (1774-1842), surgeon at the Middlesex Hospital London.

Marfan Syndrome
Congenital connective tissue disorder, characterised clinically by a tall thin individual with long limbs and digits, a high-arched palate, eye and cardiac valvular defects. Antoine Bernad-Jean Marfarn (1858 – 1942), French Paediatrician.

McBurney's Point
A point one-third of the way between the right anterior superior iliac spine and the umbilicus, under which the base of appendix is considered to most commonly be found. Charles McBurney (1845-1913), Professor of Surgery at Roosevelt Hospital, New York, USA.

Monteggia Fracture
Fracture of the proximal ulnar with dislocation of the head of the radius. Giovanni Battista Montaggia (1762-1815) Professor of Surgery, Milan.

Ottowa Ankle Rules
Guidelines developed to predict the need for x-rays in ankle trauma. Pain in the ankle, with one or more of: inability to weight bear immediately and in the emergency department, bony tenderness to the inferior six inches of the tibia or fibula posteriorly, the navicular or the base of the fifth metatarsal are indications for x-ray. If none of these are present, x-rays are not indicated.

Phalen's Manoeuvre
Full flexion of the wrist for 60 seconds causes paraesthesia in the median nerve distribution within the hand. George Phalen (1911-1988), Chief of Hand Surgery, Cleveland Clinic. President of the Association of Bone and Joint Surgeons, 1965.

Popeye's Sign
Bunching of the biceps brachii muscle, resulting in a mass in the arm due to proximal or distal biceps tendon rupture
Popeye is a fictional cartoon character who developed characteristically large biceps on ingestion of spinach.

Pouch of Douglas
Also known as the rectouterine pouch, the peritoneal pouch separating the rectum and the uterus in women, and the rectum and the bladder in men. James Douglas (1675-1742), Scottish Physician, Anatomist and Obstretrician.

Purkinje fibres
Conducting tissue of the heart spreading up from the Bundles of His throughout the ventricles. Jan Evangelista Purkinje (1787 – 1869), Professor of Physiology at Charles University, Prague.

Rigler's Sign
Also known as the double wall sign – seen on abdominal x-rays as a particularly clear outline of bowel wall, caused by air being present on both sides of the intestine in pneumoperitoneum. Leo George Rigler (1896-1979), Professor of Radiology at University of California, Los Angeles, USA.

Arch of Riolan
Also known as the meandering mesenteric artery. A vascular arcade connecting the middle colic artery with branches of the left colic. Jean Riolan (1580-1657), French Anatomist.

Pouch of Rutherford Morrison
Also known as the Hepato-Renal Pouch or Subhepatic Recess, this is the potential space between the liver and the superior pole of the right kidney, and the most dependent space in the supine abdomen. James Rutherford Morrison (1853-1939), Professor of Surgery at the University of Durham, UK.

Roux-en-Y Procedure
A surgical procedure involving two anastomoses: a gastro jejunostomy and a jejuno-jejunostomy. It looks like a letter Y, hence the name. Cesar Roux (1857-1934), Swiss Surgeon.

Scarpa's Fascia
A membranous fascial layer of the abdominal wall, superficial to the external oblique aponeurosis. Antonio Scarpa (1752-1832), Professor of Anatomy at the University of Modena, Italy.

Semon's Law of the Larynx
This states that in a progressive lesion of the recurrent laryngeal nerve, the abductors are paralysed before the adductors. This means that in incomplete paralysis the vocal cord will be in the midline, but in complete paralysis, it will be lateral. Sir Felix Semon (1849-1921), English Physician and Laryngologist.

Simmonds' Test
An examination technique performed to assess for a ruptured calcaneal tendon. The patient lies face down with their feet hanging of the bed and the calf is squeezed. No movement of the foot suggests calcaneal tendon rupture. Franklin Adin Simmonds (1911-1983), orthopaedic surgeon, Rowley Bristow Hospital.

Axillary Tail of Spence
An extension of breast tissue into the axilla. James Spence (1812-1882), Chair of Systematic Surgery at Edinburgh University.

Spigelian Hernia
A hernia through the spigelian fascia, the fascial layer between the rectus sheath and the semilunar line. Adrian van den Spiegel (1578-1625), Flemish Anatomist.

Stanford Classification
A classification system to describe site of aortic dissection. Stanford A involves the proximal thoracic aorta, with or without the distal. Stanford B is limited to the descending aorta distal to the left subclavian artery.

Suspensory Ligament of Treitz
A thin muscle that attaches the duodenal flexure to the posterior abdominal wall. This marks the division between foregut and midgut, and the retroperitoneal duodenum and intraperitoneal jejunum. Vaclav Treitz (1819-1872), Professor of Pathological Anatomy, Prague, Czechoslovakia.

Cerebral Aqueduct of Sylvius
A cerebrospinal fluid-filled space connecting the third ventricle to the fourth. Fransciscus Sylvius (1614-1672), Professor of Medicine at the University of Leiden, Holland.

Tinel's Sign
Light percussion of the median nerve within the carpal tunnel leads to tingling in the distribution of the median nerve within the hand. Jules Tinel (1879-1952), Chief of Neurology at the Hospital Henri-Rousselle, Paris.

Trendelenberg Gait
Characteristic gait associated with weak hip abductor muscles. Friedrich Trendelenburg (1844-1924), Professor of Surgery, Leipzig.

Volkmann's Contracture
Flexion contracture of the hand and wrist caused by ischaemic fibrosis of the forearm muscles. Richard von Volkmann (1830-1889) Professor of Surgery, Halle, Germany.

Weber Classification
A classification to describe position of fibula fractures in relation to the syndesmotic ligament between the distal fibula and tibia. Useful for predicting syndesmotic damage and instability of the ankle, and thus the need for operative management. Described by BG Weber in his book Die Verletzungen des Oberen Sprunggelenkes, 1972.

Wernicke's Area
Part of the superior temporal gyrus in the brain, a region involved in speech production. Carl Wernicke (1848-1905), Professor of Neurology and Pyschiatry at the University of Breslau, Austria.

1 | HEAD AND NECK

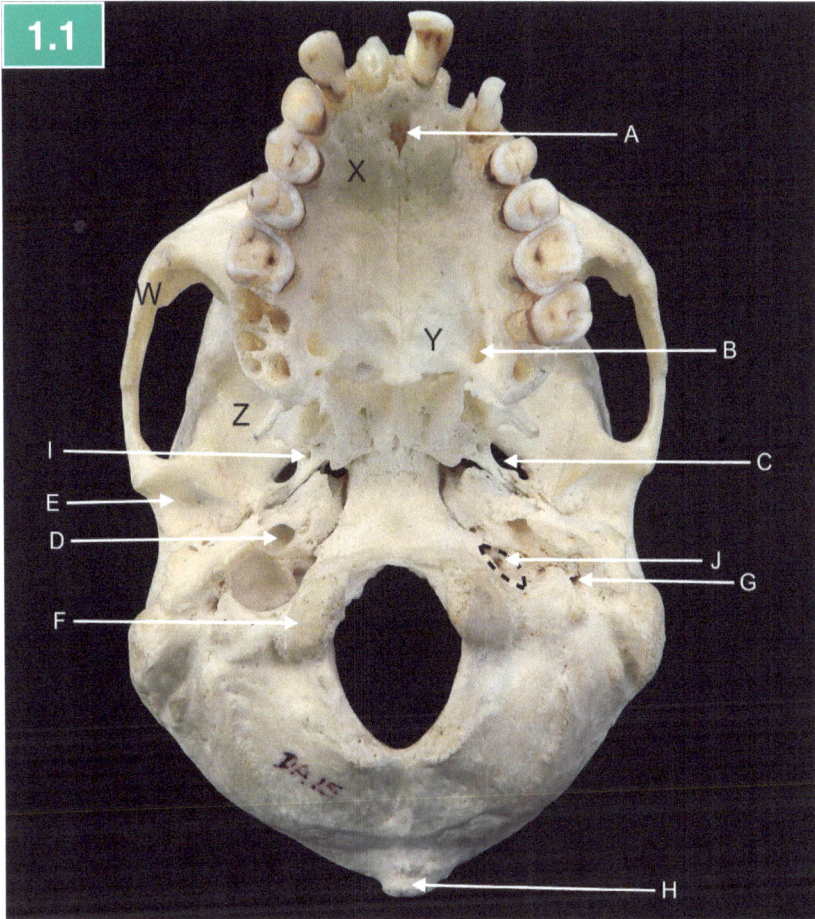

1.1

QUESTIONS

1. Name the bones W – Z.

2. Name the structures A – J.

3. Which structures pass through the jugular foramen?

4. Which structures pass through C?

5. What does J transmit?

6. Identify the foramen magnum on the specimen. Herniation of the cerebellum through here can result from severely raised intracranial pressure (ICP). Name and describe the characteristic haemodynamic response that results from raised ICP.

ANSWERS

1. W – temporal process of zygomatic bone; X –maxilla; Y – palatine bone, Z – sphenoid.

2. A – incisive fossa; B – greater palatine foramen; C – foramen ovale; D – Carotid canal; E – stylomastoid foramen; F– occipital condyles; G – stylomastoid foramen; H – external occipital protuberance; I – foramen rotundum; J – jugular foramen.

3. The jugular foramen has three compartments. The anterior compartment transmits the inferior petrosal sinus, on its way to forming the jugular vein. The intermediate transmits the glossopharyngeal (IX), vagus (X) and accessory (XI) nerves. The posterior transmits the sigmoid sinus, which joins with the inferior petrosal to form the jugular vein within the foramen.

4. The mandibular nerve (V3) and accessory meningeal artery pass through the foramen ovale.

5. The middle meningeal artery and vein and the meningeal branch of the mandibular (V3) nerve pass through the foramen spinosum.

6. Raised ICP can cause the Cushing's response, which is a rise in blood pressure to try and maintain cerebral perfusion pressure, with a compensatory bradycardia. Herniation of the cerebellar tonsils through the foramen magnum, also known as 'coning', will compress respiratory and cardiac centres in the brainstem. Paralysis will also result from spinal cord compression. This is invariably fatal if not treated and survivors are at a very high risk of residual brain damage.

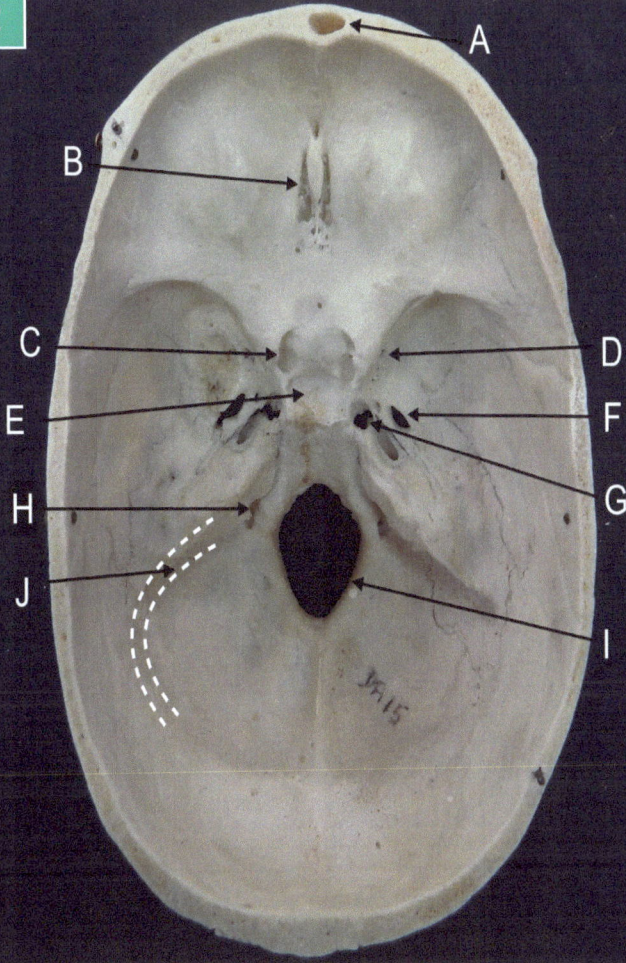

QUESTIONS

1. Identify the structures labeled A – J.

2. Through which openings do the three branches of the trigeminal pass? Name the branch and its opening.

3. The base of skull may be fractured in traumatic head injury. Name and describe some specific clinical features of this injury.

4. What passes through the hypoglossal canal? What does this supply?

5. What passes through the foramen spinosum?

6. Which bones make up the base of the skull? Demonstrate them on the specimen.

HEAD & NECK

ANSWERS

1. A – frontal sinus: B – crista galli of ethmoid bone; C – optic canal; D foramen rotundum; E – pituitary fossa; F – foramen ovale; G – internal opening of carotid canal; H – internal acoustic meatus: I – foramen magnum; J – groove for sigmoid sinus.

2. The ophthalmic branch passes through the superior orbital fissure, the maxillary branch through the foramen rotundum and the mandibular branch through the foramen ovale.

3. Signs specifically associated with base of skull fracture include CSF rhinorrhoea or otorrhoea, haemotympanum, bilateral periorbital haematomas ("raccoon eyes") and perimastoid bruising.

4. The hypoglossal nerve passes through the hypoglossal canal. It supplies all the muscles of the tongue except palatoglossus.

5. The foramen spinosum transmits the middle meningeal artery, the middle meningeal vein and the meningeal branch of the mandibular nerve.

6. The base of skull is formed by the frontal, ethmoid, sphenoid, temporal and occipital bones.

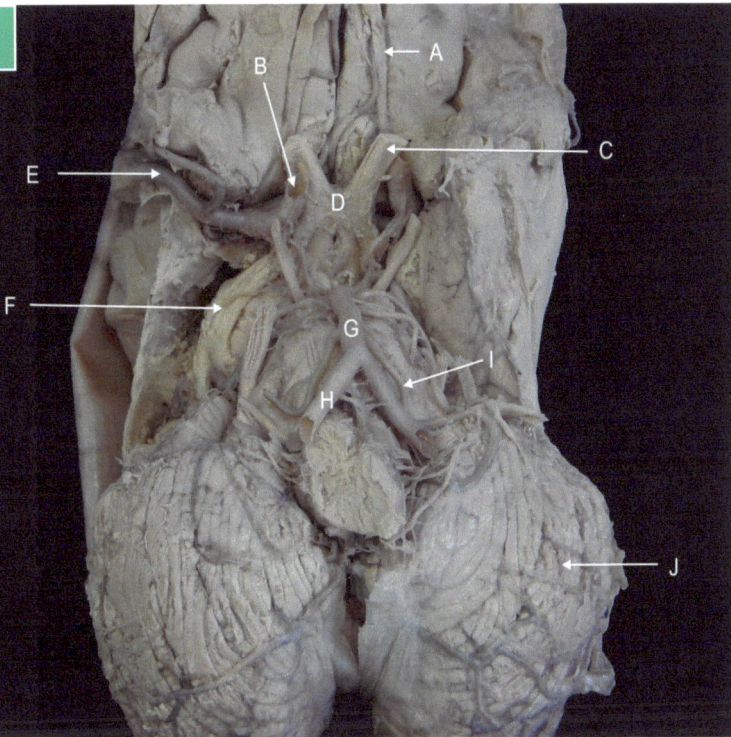

QUESTIONS

1. Name structures A – J

2. What is the origin of vessel B? Where does it penetrate the base of the skull?

3. Where is the terminal portion of the olfactory nerve found?

4. Which region of the brain is supplied by vessel E?

5. Where is the origin of the trigeminal nerve?

6. Describe the blood supply to the cerebellum.

7. What is the lateral geniculate body? Where is it found?

8. Which lobe of the brain contains the visual cortex?

9. Where may CN III be compressed if intracranial pressure is raised? How may this manifest clinically?

10. Describe the origin and course of the spinal accessory nerve from its origin to its exit from the skull.

11. Which is the only cranial nerve to pass from the posterior surface of the midbrain? How may injury to this nerve manifest clinically?

ANSWERS

1. A – olfactory nerve; B – internal carotid artery; C – optic nerve; D – optic chiasm; E – middle cerebral artery; F – optic tract; G – basilar artery; H – vertebral artery; I – anterior inferior cerebellar artery; J – cerebellum.

2. The internal carotid artery originates from the bifurcation of common carotid artery, at the level of approximately C4, and passes through the carotid canal.

3. The olfactory nerve extends to the olfactory bulb on the cribriform plate of the ethmoid bone. Multiple sensory fibres pass through the cribriform plate and provide sensory input from the nasal cavity.

4. The middle cerebral artery supplies a large region of the brain which includes the lateral surfaces of the cerebral hemispheres, excluding the superior portion of the parietal lobe and inferior portion of the temporal and occipital lobes. It has branches to the internal capsule and basal ganglia.

5. The trigeminal nerve originates from the lateral pons. It has three main branches: ophthalmic, maxillary and mandibular.

6. The cerebellum is supplied by three arteries. The superior cerebellar artery passes from the superior portion of the basilar artery, just inferior to the bifurcation of the posterior cerebral artery. The anterior inferior cerebellar artery also originates from the basilar artery. Finally the posterior inferior cerebellar artery is a lateral branch of the vertebral arteries.

7. The lateral geniculate body is a sensory relay nucleus in the thalamus. It receives approximately 90% of the optic nerve fibres from the optic tract.

8. The visual cortex is found in the occipital lobe. Axons extend from the lateral geniculate body through the optic radiation, to the visual cortex.

9. When intracranial pressure rises CN III may be compressed against the petrous part of the temporal bone. The parasympathetic fibres to the smooth muscle of sphincter pupillae are superficial and so are affected first. This leads to progressive pupillary dilation on the affected side.

10. The spinal accessory nerve originates from a series of rootlets on the lateral portions of the proximal spinal cord. These ascend through the foramen magnum into the cranial cavity and pass out through the jugular foramen together with the glossopharyngeal and vagus nerves.

11. The trochlear nerve passes from the posterior portion of the midbrain. It has a long course anteriorly around the brainstem and supplies the superior oblique muscle. If damaged it may result in diplopia worse on looking downward, for example when walking down stairs.

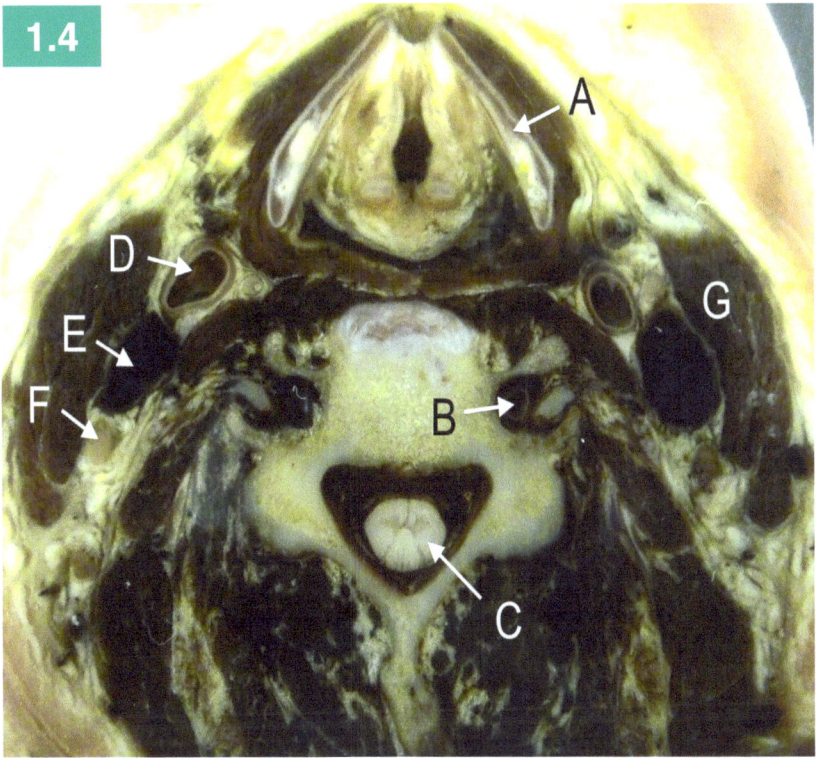

QUESTIONS

1. Name structures A – G.

2. What structures are found within the carotid sheath?

3. In addition to the carotid sheath, what other deep fascial layers are found in the neck?

4. At what level does the common carotid artery bifurcate? Which structures are found at the bifurcation? Which nerve innervates these?

5. Where are the origin and termination of the internal jugular vein?

6. How is the internal jugular vein related to the internal and common carotid arteries? What anatomical landmarks should be considered when cannulating the internal jugular vein?

ANSWERS

1. A – thyroid cartilage; B – vertebral artery in foramen tranversarium; C – spinal cord; D – common carotid artery; E – internal jugular vein; F – vagus nerve; G – sternocleidomastoid muscle

2. The carotid sheath contains the internal jugular vein, common carotid artery, vagus nerve and deep cervical lymph nodes. The ansa cervicalis is found in the wall of the sheath.

3. There are three further layers of deep fascia in the neck that all contribute to the carotid sheath. They include the pretracheal, prevertebral and investing fascia.

4. The carotid artery is frequently described as bifurcating at the level of C4, although there is wide variation. The carotid body is found at the bifurcation. It is comprised of chemoreceptors and supporting cells, as such it is sensitive to pH changes. It transmits sensory information via the glossopharyngeal nerve. Also found here is the carotid sinus, which contains baroreceptors involved in the control of blood pressure. It is innervated by branches of the glossopharyngeal nerve.

5. The internal jugular vein originates in the posterior compartment of the jugular foramen, as a continuation of the sigmoid sinus. It descends in the carotid sheath to join with the subclavian vein behind the sternoclavicular joint to form the brachiocephalic vein.

6. The internal jugular vein is initially posterior to the internal carotid artery. It then descends lateral to this vessel before becoming more anterolateral near to its termination. The centre of the triangle formed by the heads of sternocleido-mastoid and the clavicle is the point recommended for cannula insertion.

1.5

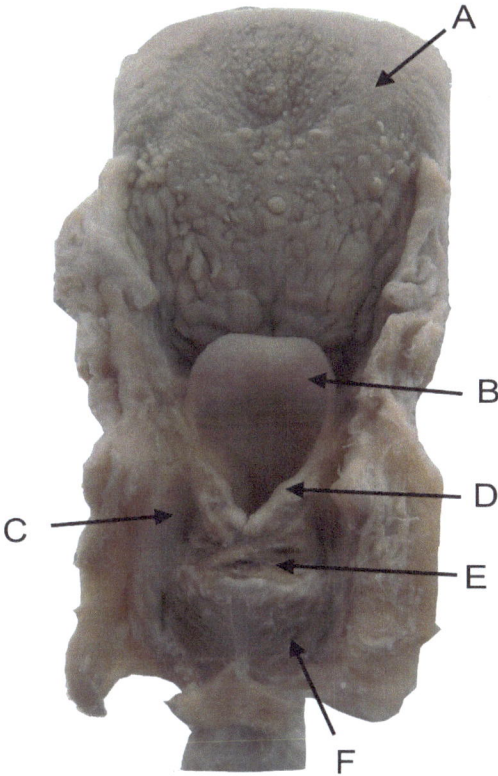

QUESTIONS

1. Identify structures A – D
2. Which muscles are represented by E?
3. What is the function of muscle F?
4. What are the boundaries of the piriform fossa?
5. What is the clinical significance of this area?
6. Describe the sensory innervation to the larynx.
7. Describe the motor innervation to the muscles of the larynx.
8. What is Semon's law?
9. Describe the blood supply to the vocal cords.
10. What structure can be found coursing through the piriform fossa?

ANSWERS

1. A – tongue; B – epiglottis; C – piriform fossa; D – aryepiglottic fold (false cords).

2. Oblique and transverse arytenoid muscles.

3. The posterior cricoarytenoid is the only intrinsic laryngeal muscle that keeps the cords abducted and therefore the patient alive.

4. Laterally is the mucosal lining of the thyroid cartilage, medially are the vocal folds, superiorly is the vallecula and inferior leads to the trachea.

5. This area is often the site of food being stuck in the larynx, typically a fish bone.

6. The sensory innervation of the larynx can be split above and below the level of the vocal cords. Above the level of the cords the internal branch of the superior laryngeal nerve is responsible for sensation. Below the level of the cords the recurrent laryngeal nerve provides the sensory innervation. Both are branches from the vagus nerve.

7. All the intrinsic muscles of the larynx are supplied by the recurrent laryngeal nerve. The only laryngeal muscle that is not supplied by this nerve is the cricothyroid muscle, which lies outside the larynx and is supplied by the external branch of the superior laryngeal nerve.

8. In a progressive lesion of the recurrent laryngeal nerve, loss of the abductor muscles will be observed before the adductor muscles.

9. The vocal cords have no submucosa and therefore receive no blood supply. They receive their nutrients from the cell secretions found in the saccule.

10. The internal branch of the superior laryngeal nerve and the superior laryngeal artery course along the piriform fossa.

1.6

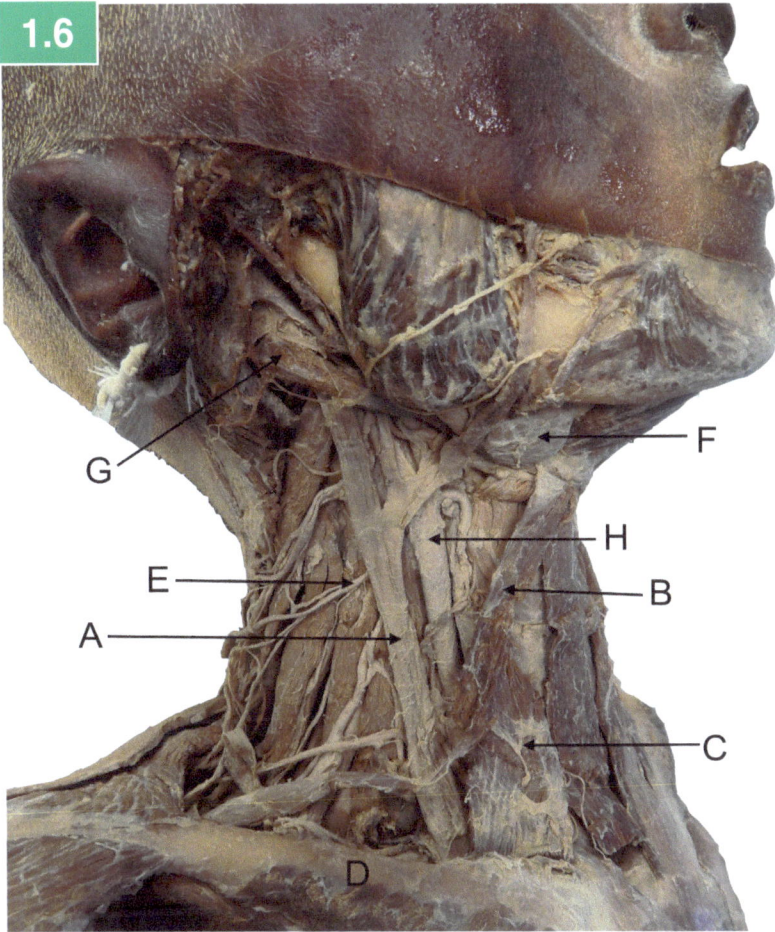

G

F

H

E

B

A

C

D

QUESTIONS

1. Name structures A – H
2. Describe the contents of the carotid sheath.
3. Where is the incision typically made to access structure F? Why is this?
4. At what vertebral levels are the hyoid bone, thyroid cartilage and carotid bifurcation?
5. What structures does E supply?
6. What is I? What is its action?

ANSWERS

1. A – internal jugular vein; B – superior belly of omohyoid muscle; C – sterno-thyroid muscle; D – clavicle; E – accessory nerve; F –submandibular gland; G – posterior belly of digastric muscle; H – carotid artery.

2. The carotid sheath contains the internal jugular vein laterally, the common and internal carotid arteries medially and the vagus nerve posteriorly. In addition deep cervical lymph nodes are found within it, and superiorly the glossopharyngeal (IX), accessory (XI) and hypoglossal nerves (XII). The ansa cervicalis is found in the anterior wall.

3. An incision to reach the submandibular gland should be made at least two fingerbreadths below the mandible, to avoid damaging the mandibular nerve or its branches.

4. The hyoid is at C2, the thyroid cartilage at C4–5 and the carotid bifurcation at the upper border of C4.

5. The accessory nerve innervates the sternocleidomastoid muscle before emerging from this muscle's posterior aspect to travel across the posterior triangle of the neck and reach the trapezius muscle, which it also supplies.

6. This is the masseter muscle. It is a powerful elevator of the mandible.

1.7

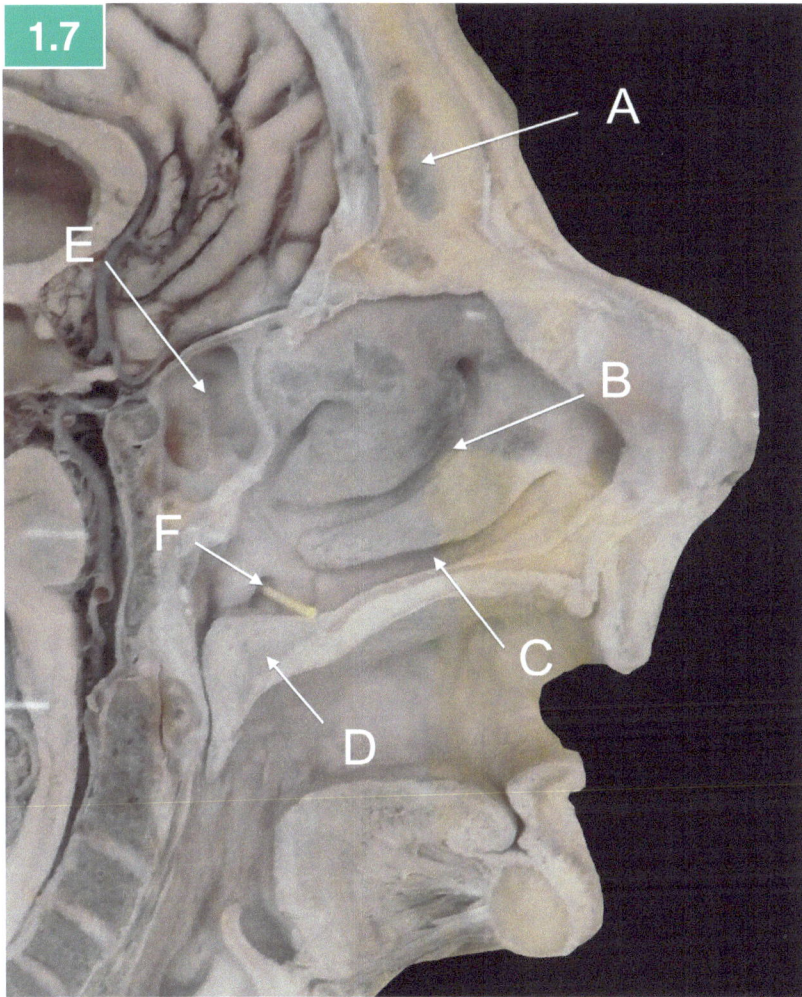

QUESTIONS

1. Identify structures A – F

2. What are the four paired nasal air sinuses?

3. Where do the frontal and maxillary air sinuses communicate with the nasal cavity?

4. What structure can be accessed through the sphenoid sinus?

5. Where is the danger triangle of the face?

6. What is the clinical relevance of the danger triangle?

ANSWERS

1. A – frontal air sinus; B – middle meatus; C – inferior meatus; D – soft palate; E – sphenoid sinus; F – pharyngotympanic tube.

2. These include the frontal, maxillary, sphenoid and ethmoidal sinuses. They surround the nasal cavity with which they communicate, via the ostia.

3. The frontal air sinus opens into the anterior middle nasal meatus. The maxillary air sinus also opens into the middle nasal meatus in a recess called the hiatus semilunaris.

4. The transphenoidal route is used to access the pituitary gland.

5. This is a triangle marked by the corners of the mouth that extends to a tip at the nasal bridge.

6. Superficial infections in this region have the potential to spread along the ophthalmic veins from the facial vein to the cavernous sinus, an effective anastomosis between facial and intracranial veins. This may lead to cavernous sinus thrombosis, meningitis or brain abscesses. This is fortunately less common following the introduction of antibiotics.

1.8

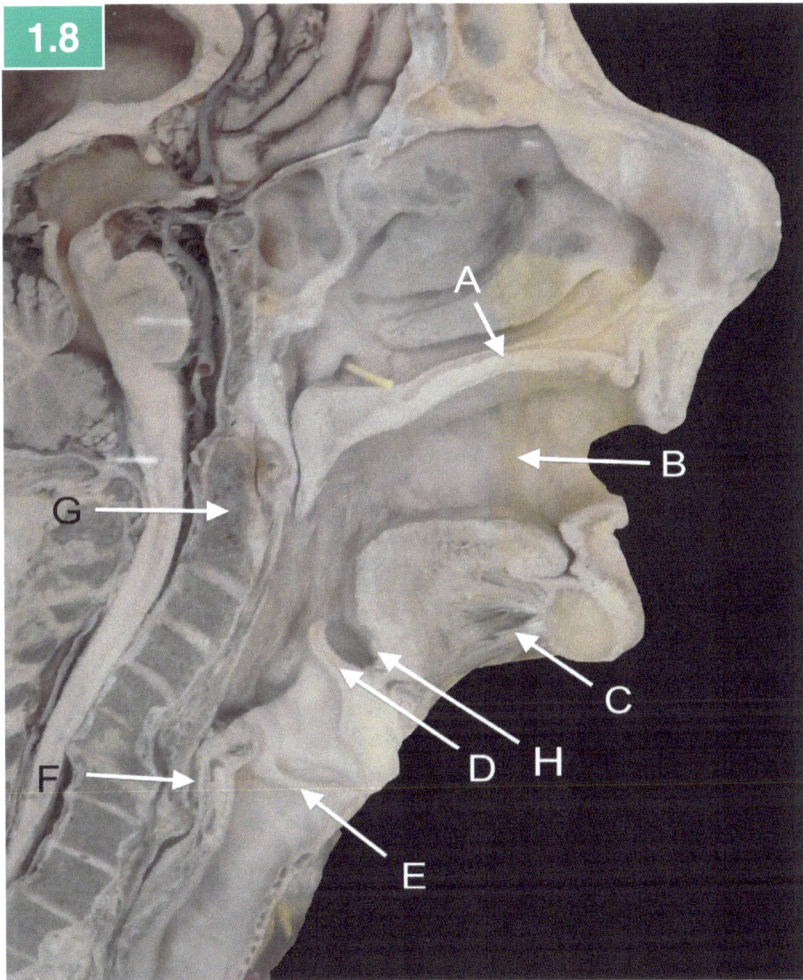

QUESTIONS

1. Identify structures A – H.

2. What are the borders of the nasopharynx?

3. Where are the pharyngeal tonsils located? What is the alternative name for them?

4. Which structures form the anterior and posterior borders of the palatine tonsils?

5. Describe the innervation of the pharynx.

6. What are the phases of swallowing? How does the pharynx contribute to this process?

7. What is Killian's dehiscence?

ANSWERS

1. A – hard palate; B – oral cavity; C – genioglossus; D – epiglottis; E – vocal folds; F – oesophagus; G – dens of C2; H – vallecula

2. This commences posterior to the nasal choanae, above the soft palate. It is bordered superiorly by the sloping base of the skull, which includes parts of the sphenoid and occipital bones.

3. The pharyngeal tonsils, also known as the adenoids, are located in the roof of the nasopharynx

4. Anterior to the palatine tonsils is the palatoglossal arch, which covers the palatoglossus muscle. This marks the boundary between the oral cavity and oropharynx. Posteriorly is the palatopharyngeal arch formed by the palatopharyngeus muscle.

5. The motor supply to the pharynx is through branches of the vagus and glossopharyngeal nerves. Branches of these nerves form the pharyngeal plexus in the pharyngeal wall.
All muscles of the pharynx are supplied by the vagus nerve except the Stylopharyngeus, which is supplied by the glossopharyngeal nerve.
The sensory innervation of the nasopharynx is by the pharyngeal branch of the maxillary nerve. Sensory supply to the oropharynx is by the glossopharyngeal nerve. Finally sensation to the laryngopharynx is supplied by the vagus nerve.

6. Swallowing is divided into oral, pharyngeal and oesophageal phases.
During the pharyngeal phase the soft palate is tensed and elevated, closing the nasopharynx. This prevents regurgitation into the nasal cavity. The base of the tongue retracts and pushes the bolus against the pharyngeal walls. The pharynx is pulled upwards and forwards, shortening its length. The oropharynx is kept closed by palatoglossus. The vocal folds close and the epiglottis tilts backwards. The upper oesophageal sphincter opens to allow passage of the bolus.

7. Killian's dehiscence is a triangular area of weakness in the inferior pharyngeal constrictor between its two parts; thyropharyngeus and cricopharyngeus muscles. This is the most likely site of pharyngeal pouch formation.

1.9

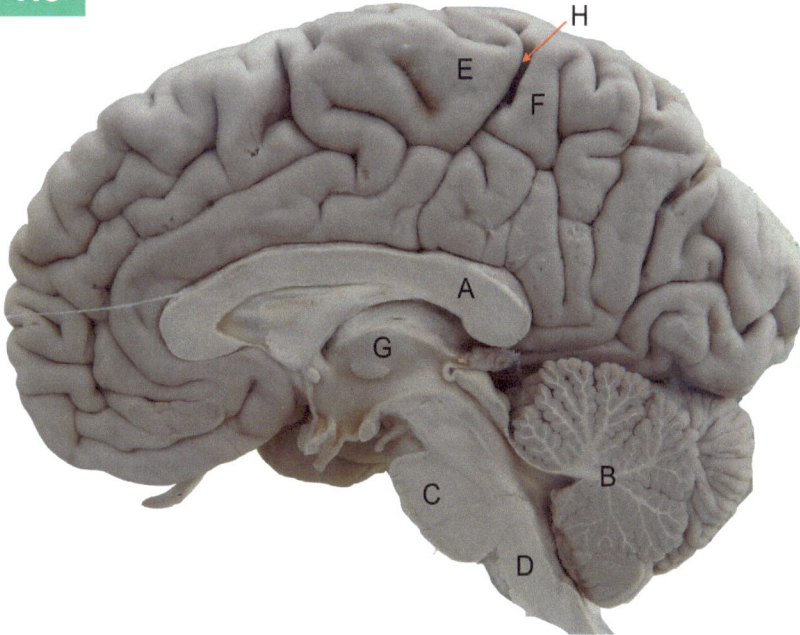

QUESTIONS

1. Name structures A – H

2. What is released from the pituitary gland?

3. What management options are available for a prolactinoma?

4. What structure separates the cerebellum from the inferior portion of the occipital lobe?

5. Where are the respiratory centers found?

6. Where is cerebrospinal fluid produced? How does it pass from the lateral ventricles to third ventricle and from the third to fourth ventricle?

7. Where are Broca's and Wernicke's areas found? Lesions here cause what typical deficits?

HEAD & NECK

ANSWERS

1. A – corpus callosum; B – cerebellum; C – pons; D – medulla; E – precentral gyrus; F – postcentral gyrus; G – thalamus; H – central sulcus

2. The pituitary gland is responsible for the release of a number of hormones. The anterior pituitary releases:

TSH	Thyroid stimulating hormone
LH	Luteinising hormone
FSH	Follicle stimulating hormone
ACTH	Adrenocorticotrophic hormone
PRL	Prolactin
GH	Growth hormone

The following hormones are released from the posterior pituitary:

OT	Oxytocin
ADH/VP	Vasopressin

3. Management options include the following:

Conservative	Watchful waiting
Medical	Dopamine agonists e.g. bromocriptine, cabergoline
Surgical	Transphenoidal pituitary surgery

4. The tentorium cerebelli is an extension of dura mater that separates the occipital lobe from the cerebellum.

5. The respiratory centres are found in the medulla. These include the inspiratory and expiratory centres. Their pattern of stimulation can be modified by the pneumotaxic and apneustic centres of the pons.

6. Cerebrospinal fluid is produced primarily by the choroid plexus of the lateral ventricles, the remainder being made by cells in the surfaces of the ventricles. It passes into the third ventricle through the interventricular foramina of Monro and via the cerebral aqueduct of Sylvius into the fourth ventricle.

7. Broca's area is found in the frontal lobe of the dominant (usually left) hemisphere of the brain. Deficiency in this region results in expressive aphasia. Wernicke's area is found in the superior temporal gyrus in the dominant cerebral hemisphere. Deficiency results in receptive aphasia.

1.10

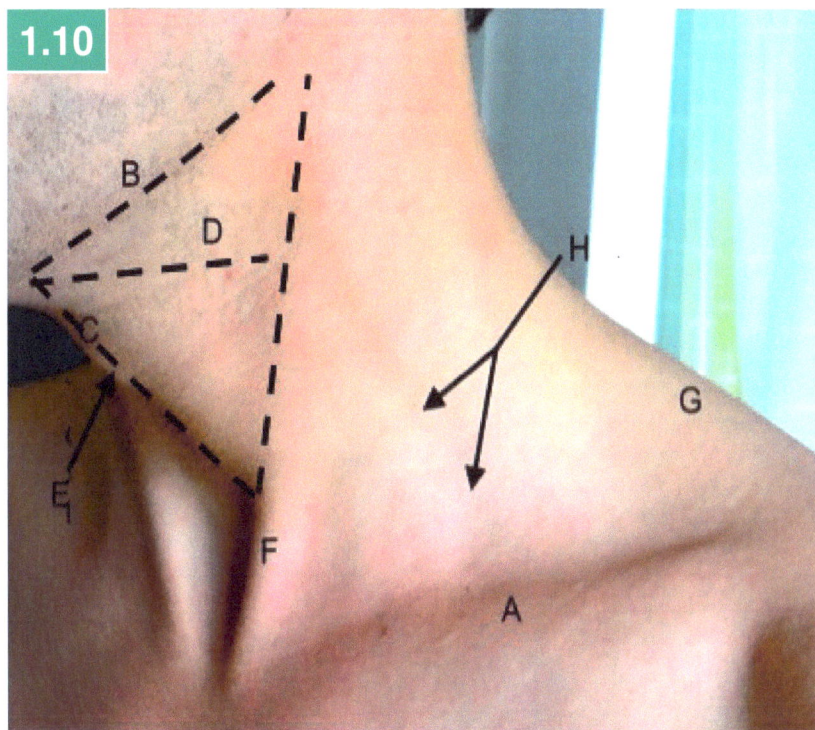

QUESTIONS

1. Name the bones A and B.
2. Which muscle is represented the line C?
3. Which anatomical triangle is represented by D?
4. Identify structures E – H.
5. What makes up the borders of the anterior and posterior triangles?
6. What is the landmark for the accessory nerve?
7. Give two ways that this nerve can be damaged.
8. Give two consequences that may result due to damage of this nerve.
9. What are the landmarks for a needle cricothyroidotomy?
10. Give two causes of a swelling in the posterior triangle of the neck.

ANSWERS

1. A – clavicle; B – mandible.

2. C – the omohyoid muscle.

3. D – submandibular triangle.

4. E – laryngeal prominence; F – sternocleidomastoid muscle; G – trapezius; H – external jugular vein.

5. The posterior triangle is formed by the superior aspect of the clavicle inferiorly, the anterior border of the trapezius muscle posteriorly and the posterior margin of the sternocleidomastoid muscle anteriorly. The anterior triangle is bound by the anterior border of the sternocleidomastoid muscle, the midline of the neck and the inferior margin of the mandible.

6. The accessory nerve can be located one–third of the distance along the posterior aspect of the sternocleidomastoid muscle from the mastoid process, passing to 5 cm above the clavicle as it enters the trapezius muscle.

7. Damage to this nerve will result in a patient being unable to shrug their shoulders on the affected side and an inability to turn one's head to the contralateral side.

8. The accessory nerve is removed deliberately in a radical neck dissection, which involves the lymphatic chain, internal jugular vein, sternocleidomastoid muscle and the spinal accessory nerve. In addition a lymph node biopsy may result in damage to this nerve.

9. A needle cricothyroidotomy can be performed by running your finger down the subject's thyroid cartilage. Once you feel the first dip you will be over the cricothyroid membrane, which is where the puncture will be made. If the clinician proceeds to move further inferiorly, they will almost immediately feel the cricoid cartilage.

10. Within the posterior triangle the most common cause of a swelling is lymphadenopathy. Two other causes may be a subclavian artery aneurysm, which will be pulsatile, and a cystic hygroma in an infant.

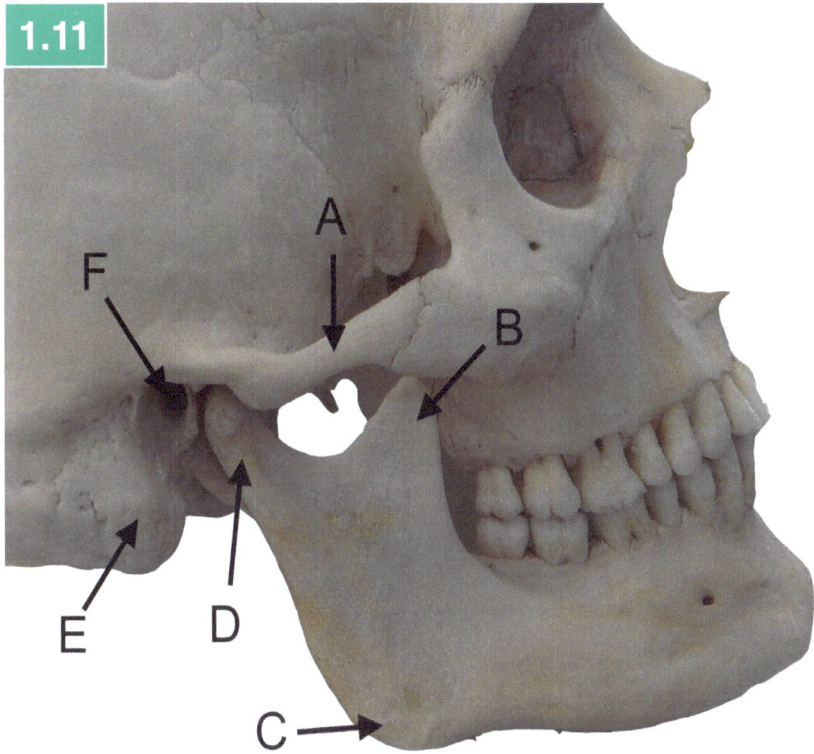

1.11

QUESTIONS

1. Label A – F.

2. Which articulating surfaces are involved in the temporomandibular joint?

3. What movements are permitted at this joint?

4. What are the boundaries of the infratemporal fossa?

5. What are the contents of the infratemporal fossa?

6. Which muscles elevate the mandible?

7. Which nerve provides sensation to the lower teeth? How is this nerve anaesthetised?

ANSWERS

1. A – zygomatic process of temporal bone; B – coronoid process of mandible; C – angle of mandible; D – mandibular condyle; E – mastoid process of temporal bone; F – external acoustic meatus.

2. The head of the mandible, which is the upper end of the condylar process, articulates with the articular fossa and articular tubercle of the temporal bone.

3. This synovial joint is completely separated into two portions by an intra–articular disc. The inferior portion permits elevation and depression of the mandible in closing and opening of the mouth. The superior portion allows protraction and retraction.

4. The borders of the infratemporal fossa are as follows:
Superior: inferior surface of the greater wing of the sphenoid and temporal bone.
Inferior: medial pterygoid muscle
Anterior: posterior surface of the maxilla
Lateral: medial border of mandible
Medial: the lateral plate of the pterygoid process anteriorly and the pharynx and muscles of the soft palate.

5. This includes the sphenomandibular ligament, medial and lateral pterygoid muscles, the maxillary artery, the mandibular nerve, branches of the facial nerve, the glossopharyngeal nerve and pterygoid plexus of veins.

6. The temporalis, masseter and medial pterygoid muscles elevate the mandible. The only muscle to depress, in addition to protruding, the mandible is the lateral pterygoid.

7. The inferior alveolar nerve innervates the lower teeth and associated gingivae. An inferior alveolar nerve block is a common procedure. The needle is inserted anterior to the arch formed by palatoglossus. The local anaesthetic is injected along the medial border of the inferior 3rd of the body of the mandible.

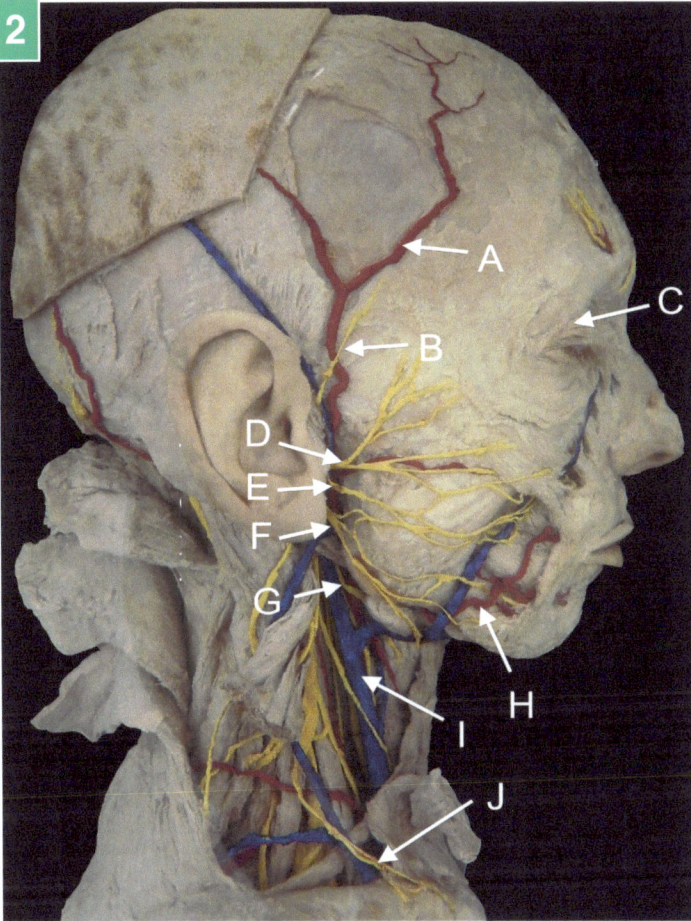

QUESTIONS

1. Identify structures A – J.

2. Which structures pass through the parotid gland?

3. Which nerve innervates the muscles of facial expression? What is its route out of the skull and what are its branches?

4. How does the parotid duct pass into the oral cavity?

5. Which parasympathetic ganglion supplies the parotid gland?

6. What is the most common type of parotid gland tumour? Which region of the parotid gland are these most commonly found?

7. During parotid gland surgery, the facial nerve may be damaged. How may this present clinically?

8. What is Frey's syndrome?

ANSWERS

1. A – superficial temporal artery; B – temporal branch of facial nerve;
C – orbicularis oculi muscle; D – zygomatic branch of facial nerve
E – buccal branch of facial nerve; F – mandibular branch of facial nerve;
G – cervical branch of facial nerve; H – facial artery; I – internal jugular vein; J –
supraclavicular nerve

2. The facial nerve, retromandibular vein, branches of the greater auricular
nerve and the external carotid artery and its distal branches.

3. The facial nerve, CN VII innervates the muscles of facial expression. It exits
the skull through the stylomastoid foramen and passes into the parotid gland.
It has 5 terminal branches that can be remembered by the mnemonic: To
Zanzibar By Motor Car. Temporal, Zygomatic, Buccal, Marginal mandibular and
Cervical.

4. The parotid duct passes anteriorly from the parotid gland, crosses the
medial border of the masseter muscle then passes into the buccal fat pad and
pierces the buccinator muscle. It opens into the oral cavity beside the second
upper molar tooth.

5. The otic ganglion.

6. Pleomorphic adenomas are the most common type of parotid gland tumour.
These benign tumours have a 1% chance of malignant change per year. Most
tumours occur in the superficial part, external to the facial nerve.

7. Damage to the temporal or upper zygomatic branches may lead to an inability
to close the eye completely. This can result in corneal dryness.
Damage to the mandibular branch can lead to weakness of the corner of
the mouth with dribbling. The corner of the mouth on the affected side is pulled
up due to the unopposed action of levator anguli oris against the denervated
depressor labii inferioris and depressor anguli oris. This may not be visible at
rest, but becomes prominent when asking the patient to smile. Damage to the
branches overall will cause paralysis of the facial muscles, including those of
the forehead.

8. During resection of the parotid gland the parasympathetic fibers that
innervate it may be damaged. As these fibres regenerate they may combine
with sympathetic nerve to the face leading to sweating when anticipating food
known as "gustatory sweating".

2 | ABDOMEN

2.1

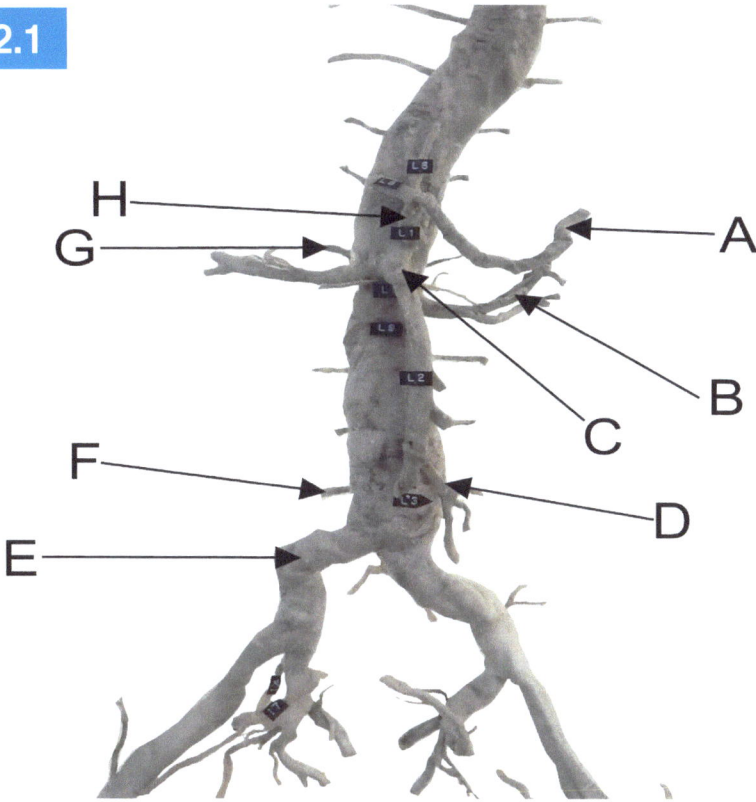

QUESTIONS

1. Identify A – H.

2. At what vertebral level does the descending aorta enter the abdomen, and what structure/s accompany it?

3. Name at least four other branches of the aorta in the abdomen.

4. At what vertebral level does the aorta bifurcate? What are the names of these branches?

5. What is the normal diameter of the aorta in the abdomen? What diameter does it have to reach to be considered aneurysmal?

6. In terms of macroscopic appearance, how may aneurysms be classified?

7. What is the difference between true and false aneurysms?

8. Describe the relationship of the inferior vena cava to the abdominal aorta.

9. Does the left renal vein pass anterior or posterior to the aorta?

ANSWERS

1. A – splenic artery; B – left renal artery; C – superior mesenteric artery; D – inferior mesenteric artery; E – right common iliac artery; F – lumber artery; G – right middle suprarenal artery; H – coeliac trunk.

2. The aorta enters the abdomen at T12. Confusingly, some texts state that it passes through the diaphragm, but it is more accurate to say that it passes behind the diaphragm, beneath the arcuate ligament between the right and left crura, just to the left of midline.

3. The branches can be classified into paired visceral (middle supra–renal, renal, gonadal); unpaired visceral (coeliac trunk, superior mesenteric, inferior mesenteric); paired parietal (inferior phrenic, 4 lumbar); and unpaired parietal (median sacral).

4. The aorta bifurcates at the level of the L4 vertebrae, just below the level of the umbilicus. It splits into the left and right common iliac arteries.

5. The normal diameter is approximately 2 cm. Aneurysms are regarded as a dilatation of a vessel 1.5 times greater than its normal diameter, so 3 cm in this case.

6. Fusiform (enlargement involving the entire diameter of the vessel) or saccular (enlargement of part of the vessel wall only, producing a balloon or sac shaped dilatation). Berry aneurysms of the cerebral circulation are classically saccular.

7. True aneurysms involve all three layers of the vessel wall (intima, media and adventitia) whereas false aneurysms involve a breach of the vessel wall allowing blood to leak out, where it is then contained by surrounding tissues. These often occur in the femoral artery due to trauma from arterial puncture, either during planned procedures such as angiography, or inadvertent arterial puncture by intravenous drug abusers. They are named false aneurysms by virtue of the fact that clinically they are felt as a pulsatile mass and so may be mistaken for true aneurysms.

8. The inferior vena cava is formed by the junction of the common iliac veins, to the right and just posterior to the aortic bifurcation, at around vertebral level L4. It passes in the retroperitoneum upwards, to the right of the aorta, moving initially from slightly posterior to anterior, before passing through the caval opening in the diaphragm at the level of T8.

9. In almost all cases, the longer left renal vein passes anterior to (over) the aorta at the level of L1. The superior mesenteric artery emerges just above it and passes anterior to the vein.

ABDOMEN

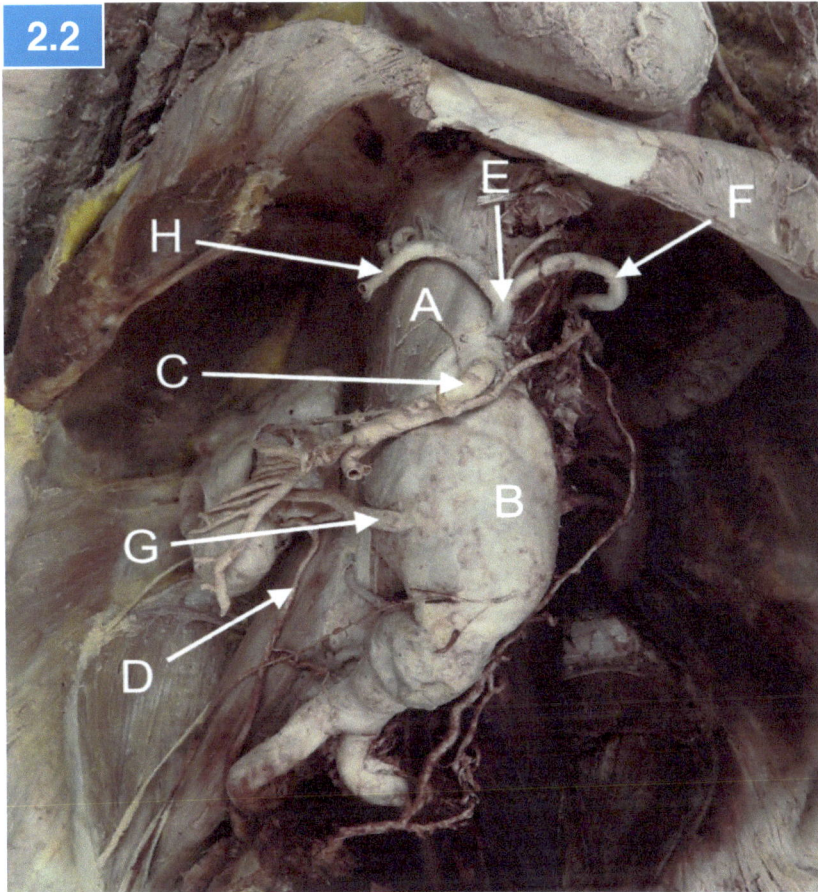

QUESTIONS

1. Name structures A – H.

2. What pathology is demonstrated here?

3. How might you classify its position with reference to major arterial branches?

4. What implications would this have for any surgical management?

5. What are the options for managing this pathology?

6. Describe some advantages and disadvantages of each type of surgical intervention.

7. When should elective operative intervention be considered?

8. Describe some risk factors for this pathology.

ANSWERS

1. A – right crus of diaphragm; B – abdominal aorta; C – superior mesenteric artery; D – right ureter; E – coeliac trunk; F – splenic artery; G – right renal artery; H – common hepatic artery.

2. This is an abdominal aortic aneurysm (AAA).

3. This is clearly suprarenal, indeed extending all the way to the diaphragm.

4. This makes repair technically more difficult, more importantly, the renal arteries need to be plumbed back into the aorta somewhere, with a graft that incorporates their origin. In addition, if performing open repair, the time the superior clamp is on has greater implications in terms of renal ischaemia.

5. This would be a technically extremely difficult repair, but broadly speaking, AAAs can be repaired by either open, laparoscopic or endovascular means (EndoVascular Aneurysm Repair – EVAR). Below 5.5 cm AAAs are traditionally monitored with ultrasound scanning.

6. Open repair is the most proven approach and is known to last for a long time, usually the patient's life. It can also deal with aneurysms too complex for endovascular repair. It does confer far greater surgical burden on the patient and so is reserved for younger, fitter patients. Laparoscopic repair is only performed in a few centres but mitigates some of the trauma of open repair, with the same advantages of open surgery. EVAR is far less invasive but does not have proven longevity (yet!) and cannot address the most complex aneurysms, though the technology is advancing all the time.

7. Any repair should be considered when the aneurysm reaches 5.5 cm in diameter. However repair is also considered if the patient is symptomatic, for example back pain or tenderness to palpation, or the aneurysm is growing at a rate greater than 0.5 cm a year.

8. Many risk factors exist for AAA; these may be classified into modifiable (smoking, alcohol use, high fat diet, hypercholesterolaemia, hypertension) and non–modifiable (age, male gender, connective tissue disease, genetic risk).

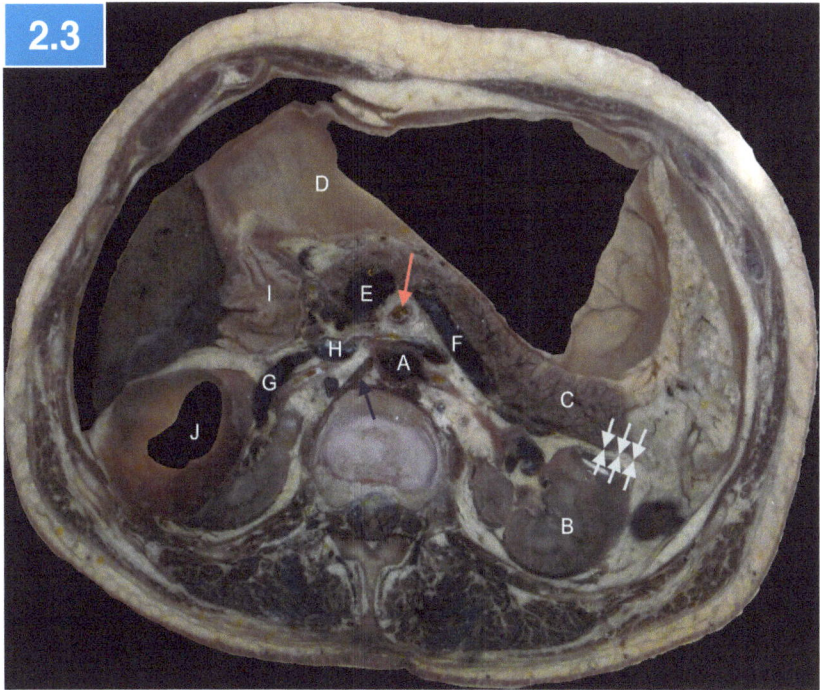

QUESTIONS

1. Name structures A – J.

2. What do the black, white and red arrows represent?

3. Where does C lie?

4. At what vertebral level does this image lie? Describe the surface landmark of this plane.

5. At what level will the coeliac, superior mesenteric, inferior mesenteric and gonadal arteries arise from the abdominal aorta?

6. Which vessels run posterior to the pancreas? What is the clinical significance of this relationship?

7. Which arteries arise from the posterior aspect of the abdominal aorta?

8. If the inferior mesenteric artery (IMA) becomes blocked how will the left side of the bowel be perfused?

9. What is Leriche's syndrome?

10. At what vertebral level will one expect to find the kidneys?

ANSWERS

1. A – abdominal aorta; B – left kidney; C – tail of the pancreas; D – antrum of the stomach; E – hepatic portal vein; F – splenic vein; G – right renal vein; H – IVC; I – second part of the duodenum; J – hepatic flexure.

2. Black arrow – right crus of the diaphragm; white arrow – perirenal fascia (of Gerota); red arrow – superior mesenteric artery (SMA).

3. The tail of the pancreas is the only part of the pancreas that is intraperitoneal; the rest of the structure is a secondary retroperitoneal structure.

4. This plane is defined as the transpyloric plane. This is the midpoint between the jugular notch and the pubic symphysis. In clinical practice this is considered a hand's breadth below the xiphoid. This is at vertebral level L1 – the prosection image is taken just below this.

5. The coeliac artery will be found at T12, SMA at L1, gonadal arteries at L2 and IMA at L3.

6. The splenic artery and vein. The vein in particular is at risk of thrombosis in episodes of severe pancreatitis.

7. These are the inferior phrenic arteries, lumbar arteries and the median sacral artery.

8. There is an anastomosis from the SMA to the IMA via the marginal artery of Drummond. This provides a collateral circulation to the left side of the bowel, allowing the vascular surgeon to oversew the IMA when repairing an AAA. Ischaemia of the left and sigmoid colon does remain a risk.

9. Leriche's syndrome is classically described as the triad of bilateral buttock and thigh claudication, absent femoral pulses and erectile dysfunction. It arises from aortoiliac occlusive disease, or a so–called saddle embolus at the aortic bifurcation.

10. The kidneys lie between the T12 and L3 vertebral levels. The right lies lower than the left, with the upper poles being protected by the floating ribs.

2.4

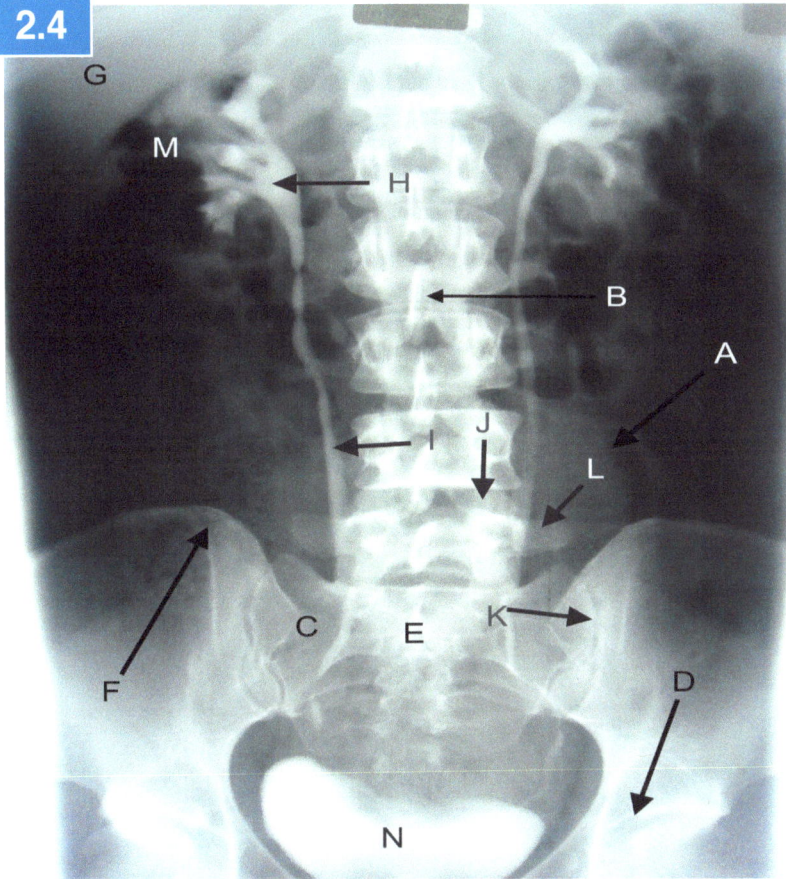

ABDOMEN

QUESTIONS

1. Name structures A – N.

2. Describe how one would differentiate between large bowel and small bowel on an abdominal radiograph.

3. What may be observed on an abdominal radiograph of a patient with a perforated viscus? What other basic imaging would help confirm the diagnosis?

4. Identify the ureters on the image. Describe and identify their possible sites of constriction.

5. Describe the typical presentation of a patient with a ureteric calculus. How may this be managed?

6. What is the blood supply to the ureters?

ANSWERS

1. A – psoas shadow; B – lumbar spinous process; C – ala of the sacrum; D – acetabulum; E – body of the sacrum; F – iliac crest; G – liver shadow; H – renal pelvis; I – ureter; J – facet joint; K – sacroiliac joint; L – transverse process of L5; M – right kidney; N – bladder.

2. The large bowel is usually found at the periphery of an abdominal radiograph and should be identified from the caecum and followed all the way around to the rectum. Characteristically it is found to have haustra, when dissected one can observe the muscular bands of taenia coli on the surface. The small bowel is found within the center of the radiograph. It possesses valvulae conniventes, which produce the appearance of bands that cross the whole width of the imaged bowel wall.

3. Air outside of the bowel wall as well as inside, producing a very clear outline of the bowel wall. This is known as Rigler's sign and suggests a pneumoperitoneum. An erect chest film may demonstrate air under the diaphragm, however this may be missing in half of cases.

4. The right ureter is shown by the letter I. Classically the ureters are constricted at three sites: the pelviureteric junction (PUJ), the vesicoureteric junction (VUJ) and the passing of the ureters over the pelvic brim. These are the usual sites for ureteric calculus impaction.

5. Ureteric calculi present with an excruciating unilateral loin to groin pain. Though in theory it is colicky, patients describe pain building up and being very severe for several hours, before it subsides (usually with the passing of a stone). If a stone remains impacted, it may occur again. Patients feel as though they need to wriggle or move to get comfortable, in contrast to those with peritonism, who wish to lie still. Examination will reveal renal angle and flank tenderness.

Management is usually conservative, with strong analgesia (usually a combination of rectal non–steroidal anti–inflammatories and opiates). Tamsulosin, an alpha–blocker, may be given to help relax the ureter. Gold–standard investigation is now a non–contrast CT scan to identify stones. Most stones pass on their own and are followed–up in clinic, but those over a certain size may require lithotripsy or surgery, typically fragmentation with a laser or ultrasound, or ureteroscopy and basket retrieval, depending on the site of impaction.

6. The ureters take a segmental blood supply from adjacent structures on their descent into the pelvis. Proximally they are supplied by branches from the renal arteries. Mid–ureters take branches from the common iliac and/or gonadal arteries. In the pelvis they are supplied by branches from the internal iliacs.

2.5

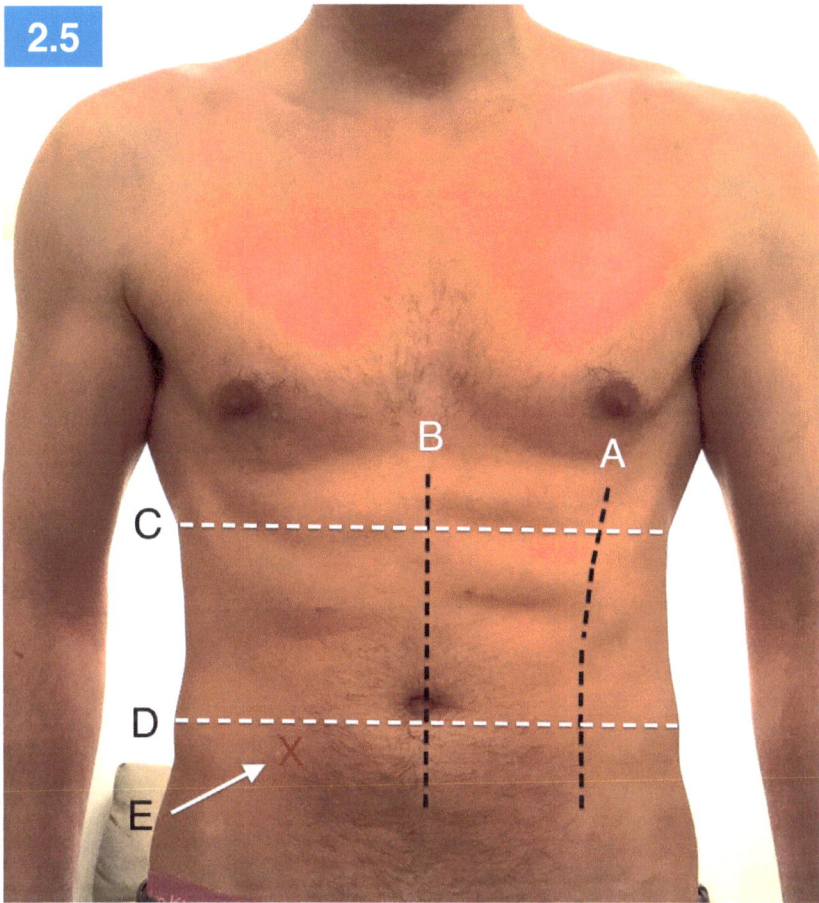

ABDOMEN

QUESTIONS

1. Name A – E.

2. Where can the fundus of the gallbladder be identified by surface land-marks?

3. Where is the spleen located?

4. Describe how a clinician may assess for hepatomegaly.

5. Where do you assess a patient for an abdominal aortic aneurysm?

6. What structure may be found at E?

7. Where should a doctor place his stethoscope to listen for renal bruits?

8. Describe the surface markings of the liver.

ANSWERS

1. A – linea semilunaris; B – linea alba; C – transpyloric line; D – transtubercular line; E – McBurney's point.

2. The fundus of the gall bladder will be located at the tip where the right linea semilunaris will come into contact with the costal margin. This is at the tip of the ninth rib.

3. The spleen lies on the posterolateral aspect of ribs 9–11 on the left side of the ribcage.

4. The liver enlarges from the right hypochondrium to the right iliac fossa. An enlarged liver is suggested to be two finger's breadths below the costal margin, therefore it is important to assess from the right iliac fossa upwards.

5. This can be assessed by placing the radial border of each index finger over the midline, above the umbilicus. An aneurysm will be both pulsatile and expansile.

6. At McBurney's point one may be palpating over the base of the appendix, although the position of the appendix is highly variable. This point is two–thirds of the way from the umbilicus to the ASIS. The most common positions of the appendix is retrocaecal but it can also be preileal, postileal or pelvic.

7. Renal bruits can be heard over the renal arteries, which are found two inches above and lateral to the umbilicus.

8. The liver margins are found between the fourth rib, anteriorly, on the right, extending to 2 cm below the costal margin and extending to the 5th intercostal space at the midclavicular line on the left side.

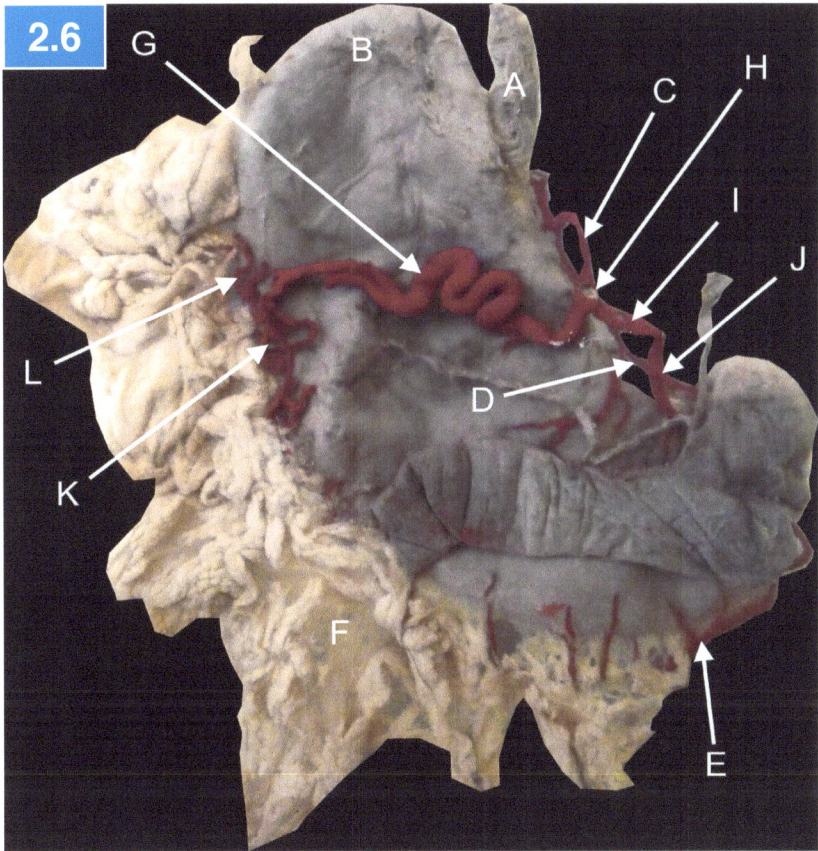

ABDOMEN

QUESTIONS

1. Name A – G on this view of the stomach from its posterior aspect.

2. At which vertebral level is the coeliac axis found?

3. What is at risk from an ulcer eroding through the posterior wall of the stomach?

4. What vessel is at risk from an ulcer eroding through the posterior wall of the first part of the duodenum?

5. When performing an oesophago–gastro–duodenoscopy (OGD), which area on the lesser curvature should the endoscopist ensure they examine?

6. Describe the blood supply to the pancreas.

7. What are the potential long–term consequences of a splenectomy? What measures can be taken to mitigate these risks?

ABDOMEN

ANSWERS

1. A – oesophagus; B – fundus; C – left gastric artery; D – right gastric artery; E – right gastroepiploic artery; F – greater omentum; G – splenic artery; H – coeliac trunk; I – common hepatic artery; J – gastroduodenal artery; K – left gastroepiploic artery; L – short gastric arteries.

2. This is found at T12 as soon as the abdominal aorta passes beneath the crura of the diaphragm.

3. An ulcer eroding through the posterior wall of the stomach may erode through the splenic artery and cause a profuse arterial bleed.

4. An erosion through the posterior wall of the first part of the duodenum may erode through the gastroduodenal artery as this courses behind it.

5. The clinician should always ensure that they assess the angular incisure, which is located in the lesser curvature close to the pylorus. Pathology in this area is easily missed.

6. The pancreas overlies the splenic vessels. Its blood supply is complex. The head is supplied by the superior and inferior pancreaticoduodenal arteries; the neck, body and tail by branches from the splenic artery.

7. Splenectomy for trauma is commonly performed, though sometimes preservation surgery may be undertaken, if possible. Removal of the spleen places the patient at risk of Overwhelming Post–Splenectomy Sepsis (OPSS), which is caused mainly by encapsulated organisms. For this reason, the patient should be vaccinated for Haemophilus Influenza B (HiB), Streptococcus Pneumoniae and Neisseria Meningitides. The patients are usually recommended to take prophylactic Penicillin V for life and carry a "Medicalert" card. Splenectomy otherwise has minimal effects on life; these include a high platelet and leukocyte count, and the presence of Heinz or Howell–Jolly bodies in the blood.

2.7

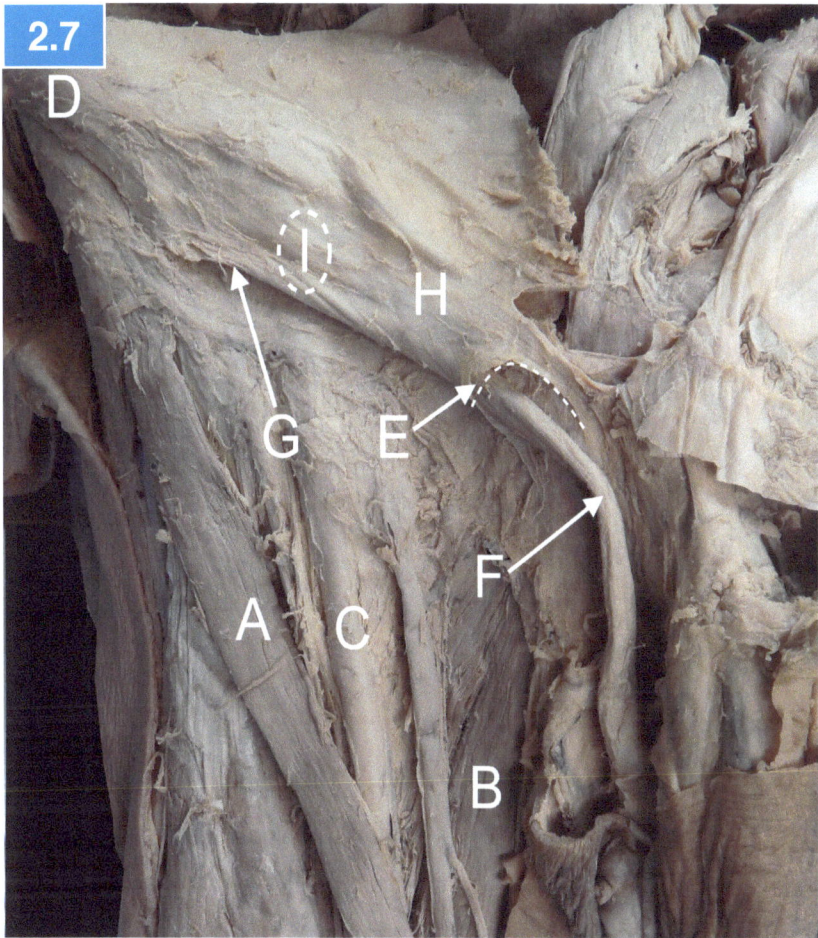

ABDOMEN

QUESTIONS

1. Name structures A – I.

2. Define the anatomical difference between a direct and indirect hernia.

3. What are the anatomical boundaries that define a lumbar hernia?

4. What are the differential diagnoses of swellings in the femoral triangle?

5. What will an air–fluid level on a chest radiograph suggest?

6. In a patient complaining of pain and a swelling lateral to the rectus abdominis muscle, what may be the cause?

7. Describe the clinical features that can be attributed to a swelling in the scrotum suggestive of an inguinoscrotal hernia.

ANSWERS

1. A – sartorius; B – adductor longus; C – femoral artery; D – ASIS; E – superficial inguinal ring; F – spermatic cord; G – inguinal ligament; H – external oblique fascia; I – deep inguinal ring.

2. A direct hernia is one where abdominal contents herniate through a weakening in the anterior abdominal wall. It will herniate through an area called Hasselbach's triangle. The borders include the inguinal ligament inferiorly, the linea semilunaris medially and the inferior epigastric artery laterally. An indirect hernia is herniation through the inguinal canal. If the hernia stops short of exiting the superficial ring, the swelling may be confused with a direct hernia.

3. This type of hernia is found in the lumbar triangle, on the back of a subject. The boundaries include the latissimus dorsi medially and external oblique laterally, with the iliac crest inferiorly.

4. Swelling in this region can be a femoral hernia, a saphenavarix (4cm below and lateral to the pubic tubercle), Cloquet's node or an aneurysm (true or false). Femoral hernias will emerge below and lateral to the pubic tubercle whereas an inguinal hernia will be above and medial. The femoral canal includes the inguinal ligament anteriorly, pectineal ligament posteriorly, lacunar ligament medially and femoral sheath laterally. Due to the tight space a hernia in this region is likely to strangulate.

5. An air–fluid level on chest radiograph would suggest stomach herniating through the oesophageal hiatus into the thorax. This can be either a sliding or rolling hiatus hernia, which may need surgical repair if medical treatment has been exhausted and the patient is still symptomatic.

6. The rectus muscles form the anterior two–thirds of the anterior abdominal wall. At the edge of the rectus is the linea semilunaris. If a weakening occurs at this region, bowel may herniate through the linea semilunaris, forming a Spigelian hernia. Differentials include a rectus sheath haematoma or a lipoma.

7. The features include bowel sounds being present in the scrotum, not being able to get above the mass, swelling separate to the testis and failure to transilluminate.

2.8

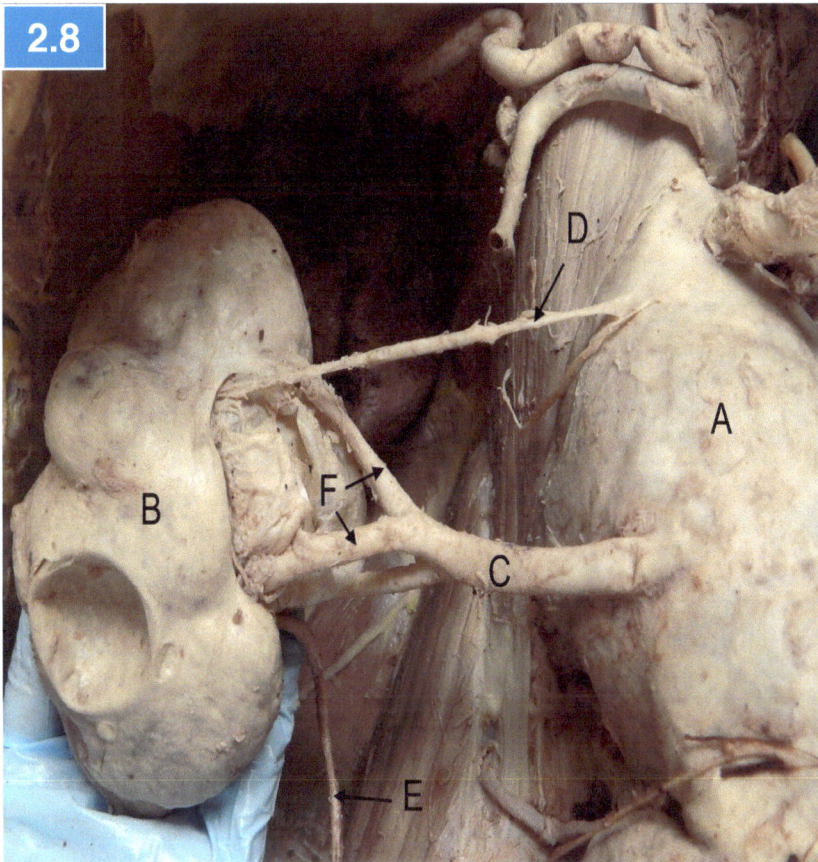

ABDOMEN

QUESTIONS

1. Name structures A – F.

2. At what height are the kidneys found on the posterior wall of the abdomen? Are they intraperitoneal or retroperitoneal organs?

3. What structures are associated with the anterior surface of the right kidney?

4. How many segments does each kidney have?

5. Describe the venous drainage of the kidneys.

6. Describe possible variation in the arterial supply to the kidney.

7. In renal trauma, how may the severity of renal injury be graded?

ANSWERS

1. A – abdominal aorta (aneurysmal in this specimen); B – right kidney; C – renal artery; D – accessory renal artery; E – ureter; F – anterior and posterior divisions of renal artery.

2. The kidneys are retroperitoneal organs. They are enclosed in perinephric fat, which is surrounded by the extraperitoneal renal fascia. The right kidney is slightly lower than the left, due to the presence of the liver. The kidneys extend from approximately T12 to L3.

3. From superiorly to inferiorly the structures associated with the anterior surface of the kidney are as follows: right suprarenal gland, liver, descending part of duodenum, right colic flexure, loops of small bowel.

4. Each kidney can be separated into 5 segments, each with its own arterial supply. These are the apical, upper anterior, middle anterior, lower and posterior segments.

5. The renal veins form in the renal sinus. They lie anterior to the renal arteries and drain into the inferior vena cava at the level of L2. The left renal vein is longer than the right and passes anterior to the abdominal aorta.

6. During the 6th to 9th weeks of fetal development the kidneys ascend from their origin in the pelvis to their final position on the posterior abdominal wall. During this ascent the kidneys receive their blood supply from a series of transient renal arteries from the abdominal aorta. Incomplete degeneration of these vessels may lead to abnormal patterns of renal arteries, which include an additional vessel to the upper pole, lower pole or two or more individual renal arteries.

7. The American Association for the Surgery of Trauma (AAST) describes five grades of renal injury. Grade 1 is a contusion or non–expanding subscapular haematoma. Grade 2 is a laceration less than 1 cm, Grade 3 a laceration greater than 1 cm, without renal pelvic involvement. Grade 4 involves damage to the collecting system, segmental infarction, urine extravasation or contained vascular injury, and Grade 5 involves a shattered kidney or renal pedicle avulsion.

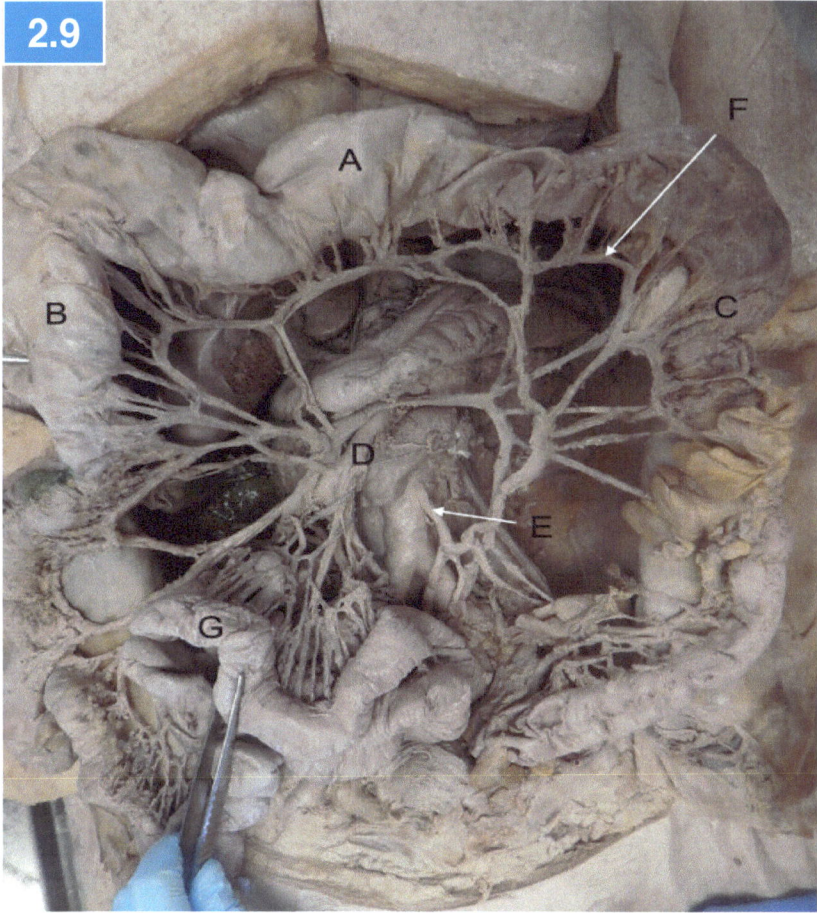

ABDOMEN

QUESTIONS

1. Identify structures A – G.

2. What features distinguish the large intestine from small intestine?

3. What anatomical structures make up the large intestine?

4. Describe the vascular supply to the appendix.

5. What is the marginal artery (of Drummond)?

6. Which regions of the colon are intraperitoneal?

7. Where does the rectum commence?

8. Describe the Dukes' stages of carcinoma of the large bowel.

9. How may full and partial–thickness rectal prolapses be differentiated clinically?

ANSWERS

1. A – transverse colon; B – ascending colon; C – descending colon;   D – superior mesenteric artery; E – inferior mesenteric artery; F – marginal artery of Drummond; G – ileum.

2. Features specific to the large bowel include:
• Comparatively broader internal and external diameter
• Contains haustrations – sacculations in the wall of the colon
• Taenia coli – 3 longitudinal bands of smooth muscle. Tonic contraction of this muscle produces the haustration of the large bowel
• Omental appendices, fat filled tags are found on the surface of the colon.

3. The large intestine comprises the caecum, appendix, ascending, transverse, descending and sigmoid colon, rectum and anal canal

4. The appendix is supplied by the appendicular artery, a branch of the ileocolic artery, which originates from the SMA. It passes into the mesoappendix and runs near its free margin. Venous drainage passes along the appendicular vein, to the ileocolic vein and into the SMV.

5. The marginal artery is a series of anastamotic arcades between branches of the SMA and IMA.

6. The caecum, transverse and sigmoid colon are intraperitoneal. The root of the transverse mesocolon passes along the inferior border of the pancreas. The transverse colon has a very variable position in the abdominal cavity.
The line of attachment of the sigmoid mesocolon is an inverted V shape on the posterior pelvic wall. Rotation of the sigmoid colon on this mesentery leads to sigmoid volvulus.

7. The true site at which the rectum forms is subject to much debate in the rectal cancer literature. It is best regarded as the site at which the three taeniae coli coalesce to form the single muscular wall of the rectum.

8. In 1932 Cuthbert Dukes described 3 stages of colorectal cancer: A, B and C. Stage D was later added.

A	Confined to mucosa
B	Extending to muscularis mucosa
C	Regional lymph node involvement
D	Distant metastasis

9. This can be difficult clinically. Full thickness rectal prolapse will feature circumferential folds, whereas a mucosal or partial–thickness prolapse will have radial folds.

ABDOMEN

2.10

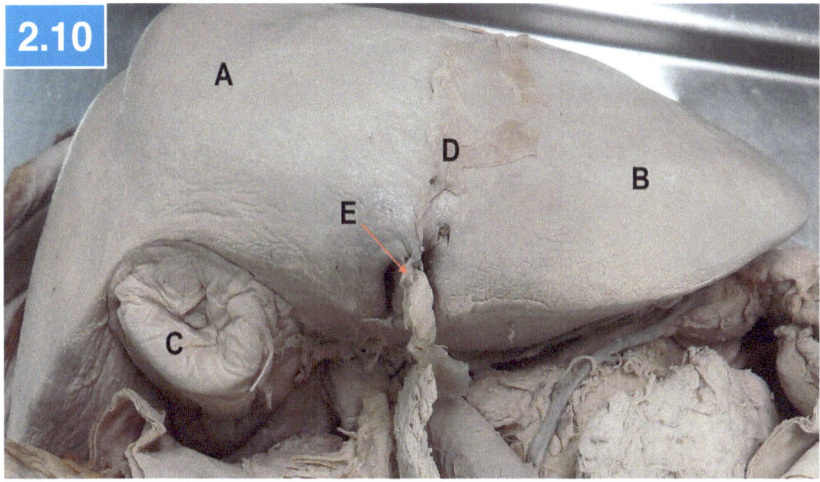

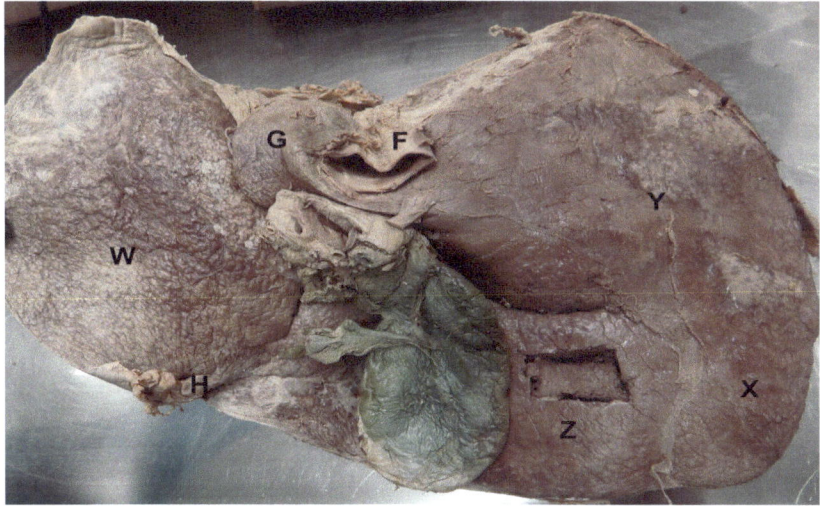

QUESTIONS

1. Identify A – E.

2. E is a vestigial remnant of which fetal structure?

3. What is the surface marking for C?

4. What are the constituents of the portal triad? Describe their orientation and its location.

5. What is Calot's triangle? What is its significance?

6. Identify F – H.

7. Identify the structures that produce the impressions marked W – Z.

8. Why is the hepatorenal pouch clinically important?

ANSWERS

1. A – right lobe of liver; B – left lobe of liver; C – fundus of gallbladder; D – falci-form ligament; E – ligamentum teres (round ligament).

2. The fetal umbilical vein degenerates to form the round ligament in the adult.

3. The fundus of the gallbladder is located in the transpyloric plane in the midclavicular line. The transpyloric plane is halfway between the jugular notch and the symphysis pubis, at the level of L1. This is considered to be a hands–breadth below the xiphoid process. Many structures lie in this plane, including the termination of the spinal cord, the origin of the superior mesenteric artery, the body of the pancreas, fundus of the gallbladder, first part of the duodenum and the duodenojejunal (DJ) flexure.

4. The portal triad consists of the hepatic artery, portal vein and the common bile duct. It is found in the free edge of the lesser omentum, also known as the hepatoduodenal ligament. The artery is medial, the bile ducts lateral and the portal vein posterior.

5. Calot's (cystohepatic) triangle is formed by the cystic duct laterally, the undersurface of the liver superiorly and the common hepatic duct medially. It is important during surgery on the gallbladder as the cystic artery (which must be clipped and divided) is found within the triangle. A single lymph node, Lund's node, may also be found here.

6. F – inferior vena cava; G – caudate lobe; H – falciform ligament.

7. W – gastric impression X – colic impression; Y – renal impression; Z – duode-nal impression.

8. The hepatorenal pouch (pouch of Rutherford–Morrison) is important because it is the most dependent (lowest) area of the peritoneum when the person is ly-ing supine. As such, fluid such as pus may accumulate here.

2.11

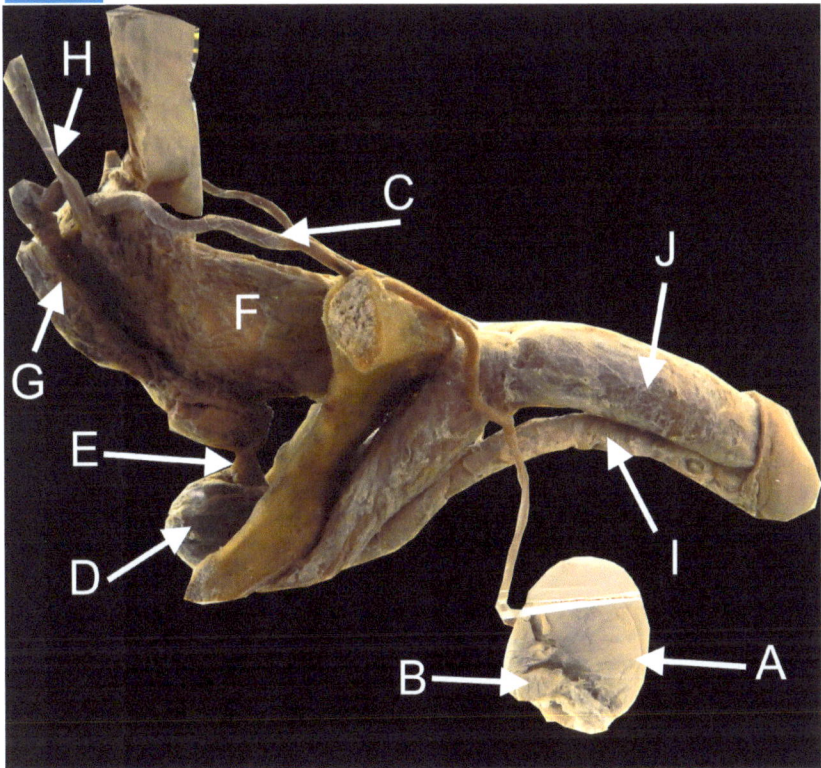

QUESTIONS

1. Label A – J.

2. Why are metastatic deposits from prostate cancer commonly found in the spine?

3. Why will stimulating the thigh elicit the cremasteric reflex?

4. What is the continuation of Scarpa's fascia that surrounds the root of the penis and the scrotum?

5. To which nodes do prostate cancers usually spread?

6. What part of the nervous system is responsible for erection and ejaculation? How does the sympathetic nervous system act in response to bladder filling and how is this beneficial during ejaculation?

7. Which structure should the urologist specifically identify during a TURP procedure?

ANSWERS

1. A – testis; B – epididymis; C – vas deferens; D – prostate; E – urethra; F — bladder; G – seminal vesicle; H – ureter; I – corpus spongiosum; J – corpus cavernosum.

2. The deep pelvis has a very rich venous supply that is in continuation with the venous drainage of the spinal canal. The network is called the vertebral venous plexus of Batson. This provides an easy route of spread for cancers of the pelvic organs to the spinal bones.

3. The cremasteric reflex is controlled by the genitofemoral nerve. The nerve is part of the lumbar plexus, which arises from the L1 and L2 nerve roots. It pierces the psoas major muscle to give of two branches; a sensory femoral branch to the area of the thigh over the femoral triangle and a motor branch to the cremasteric muscle.

4. Scarpa's fascia is the connective tissue fascia of the abdominal wall. It continues down into and around the root of the penis as Buck's fascia, which is in turn surrounded by dartos fascia. Dartos fascia will continue into the scrotum and as it reaches the perineum it will continue as Colle's fascia.

5. The prostate drains into the internal iliac veins. As a general rule, lymphatic drainage follows the venous drainage. Therefore the lymphatic vessels drain to the internal iliac nodes and may pass to sacral nodes in addition.

6. The Parasympathetic Points (erection) and the Sympathetic nervous system Shoots (ejaculation). The sympathetic nervous system is responsible not only for peristalsis of the vas and ejaculatory duct but is also responsible for contraction of the internal urethral sphincter. Therefore this will stop retrograde ejaculation and inhibit the passing of urination if socially unacceptable.

7. During a transurethral resection of the prostate (TURP) procedure the urologist must identify an area called the verumontanum or seminal colliculus. This elevated ridge contains the prostatic utricle. If the urologist ventures below this point there may be damage to the external urethral sphincter, leading to incontinence.

2.12

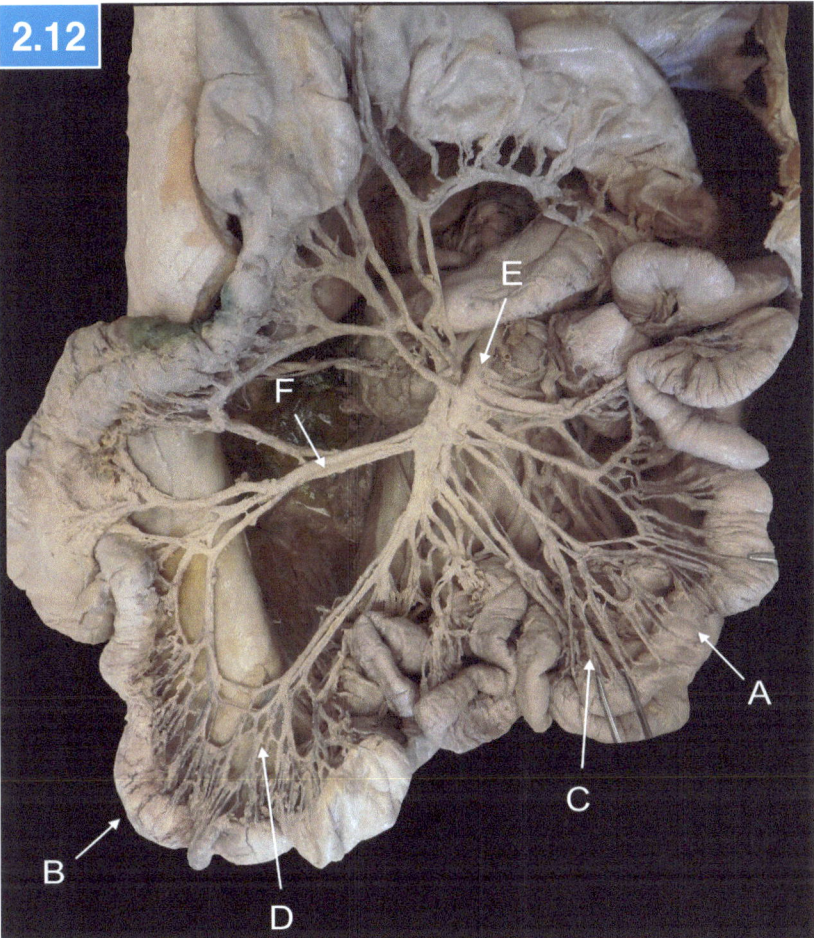

QUESTIONS

1. Identify images A – F.

2. What are the characteristic macroscopic features of the ileum?

3. At what vertebral level does the small bowel begin?

4. What is this plane called? What other structures are found at this level?

5. Which regions of the small bowel are intraperitoneal? Which are retro-peritoneal?

6. Describe the arterial supply to the small bowel.

7. What are the most common causes of small bowel obstruction?

ANSWERS

1. A – jejunum; B – ileum; C – vasa recta; D – arterial arcades; E – superior mesenteric artery; F – ileocolic artery and vein.

2. The ileum is characterized by high vascularity with short vasa recta and multiple small loop arterial arcades. The wall is thin and light with a paler pink appearance.

3. The duodenum begins at the pylorus at the level of L1.

4. The transpyloric plane. This plane, midway between the jugular notch and pubic crest includes:
   • Pylorus of the stomach
   • Duodenojejunal (DJ) flexure
   • Fundus of the gallbladder
   • Body of the pancreas
   • Origin of the superior mesenteric artery
   • Termination of the spinal cord
   • Hila of the kidneys
   • Origin of portal vein
   • Hilum of the spleen

5. The jejunum and ileum are both intraperitoneal. The root of their mesentery passes obliquely, inferiorly and to the right from the duodenojejunal junction to the ileocolic junction. The majority of the duodenum is retroperitoneal apart from the first 2 cm of the first part.

6. The duodenum is supplied by arteries that arise from the coeliac trunk via the gastroduodenal artery, and superior mesenteric artery via the inferior pancreato-duodenal artery. Branches of the superior mesenteric artery supply the jejunum and ileum.

7. The most common cause of small bowel obstruction is adhesions, usually relating to previous surgery. Causes may be usefully classified into intraluminal (gallstone ileus, bezoar, faecal impaction, foreign body); intramural (cancer, stricture) and extraluminal or external (adjacent mass causing compression, adhesions, herniation).

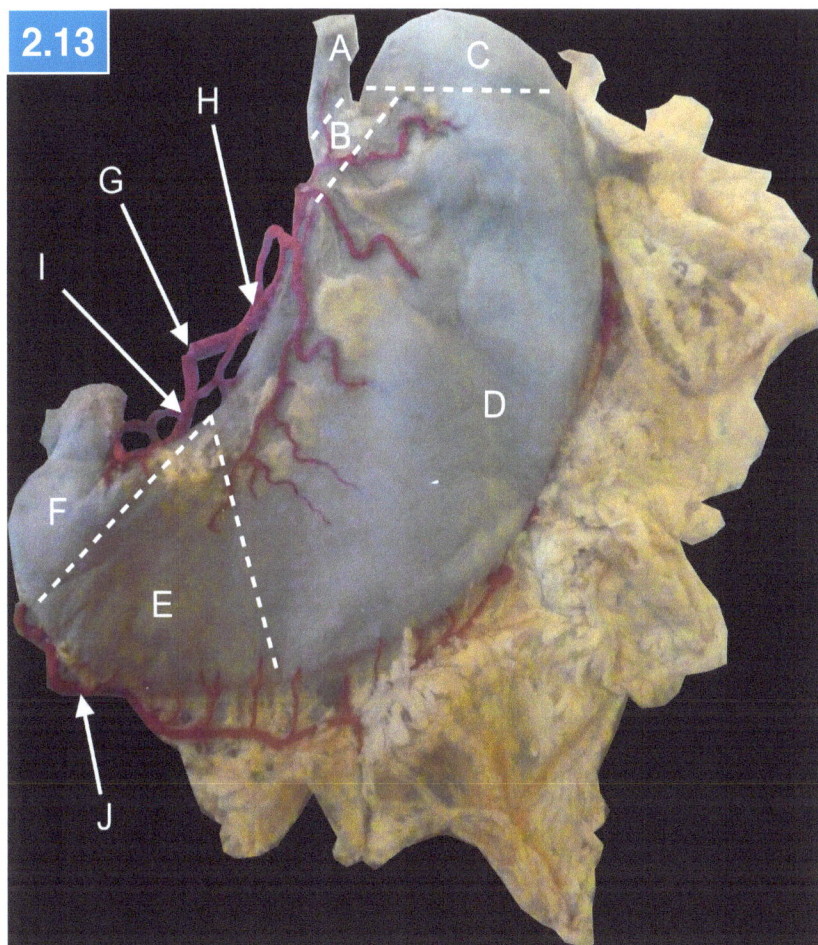

QUESTIONS

1. Identify A – J.

2. Of which artery is J a branch?

3. What is the significance of the artery identified in question 2 to peptic ulcer disease?

4. What is Barrett's oesophagus? Describe the different cell types involved

5. What is the most common aetiological agent in the pathogenesis of duodenal ulcers? How may it be treated?

6. Describe some "red flag" symptoms in a patient with dyspepsia that increase the suspicion for gastric cancer.

7. How may gastric cancer be managed?

ANSWERS

1. A – oesophagus; B – cardia; C – fundus; D – body; E – antrum; F – pylorus; G – coeliac trunk; H – left gastric artery; I – common hepatic artery; J – right gastroepiploic artery.

2. The right gastroepiploic artery is a terminal branch of the gastro–duodenal artery.

3. The gastroduodenal artery is the most common source of arterial bleeding in posterior duodenal ulcers.

4. Barrett's oesophagus is intestinal metaplasia of the distal oesophagus. Repeated exposure to acidic gastric contents causes the normal stratified squamous epithelium of the oesophagus to be replaced by simple columnar epithelium normally found in the stomach. This is considered a pre–malignant process, with an approximate 50–fold increased risk in oesophageal cancer.

5. Colonisation of the stomach and duodenum by Helicobacter Pylori is found in over 90% of cases of duodenal ulcer. It is treated by a regime of a high dose proton pump inhibitor and two antibiotics, e.g. Lansoprazole 30mg BD in combination with Amoxicillin 1g BD and Clarithromycin 500mg BD.

6. Gastric cancer often presents late and non–specifically. The main feature is typically dyspepsia, making diagnosis difficult. Red flag features include continuous dyspepsia of less than 12 months duration in a patient older than 55; weight loss; anaemia; anorexia; and presence of risk factors, such as pernicious anaemia, previous peptic ulcer surgery, atrophic gastritis, intestinal metaplasia and first–degree relative with gastric cancer.

7. Gastric cancer is treated primarily by surgery, either curative or palliative, depending on stage. The type of operation depends on the location of the tumour. Traditionally, distal tumours are treated with a subtotal gastrectomy, with either loop or Roux–en–Y gastro–jejunostomy. Proximal tumours require total gastrectomy with oesophago–jejunostomy. There is debate over how extensive a lymphadenectomy to should be. More extensive lymphadenectomy to include the nodes surrounding the arterial supply of the stomach (D2 lymphadenectomy) is popular particularly in Japan, but may not offer a survival benefit.

Superficial tumours can be treated with endoscopic mucosal resection (EMR) or endoscopic submucosal dissection (ESD). Chemotherapy is of limited utility but is often given neo–adjuvantly to try and shrink the tumour prior to resection. Radiotherapy is also used adjuvantly. Palliative procedures include bypassing or stenting the tumour.

2.14

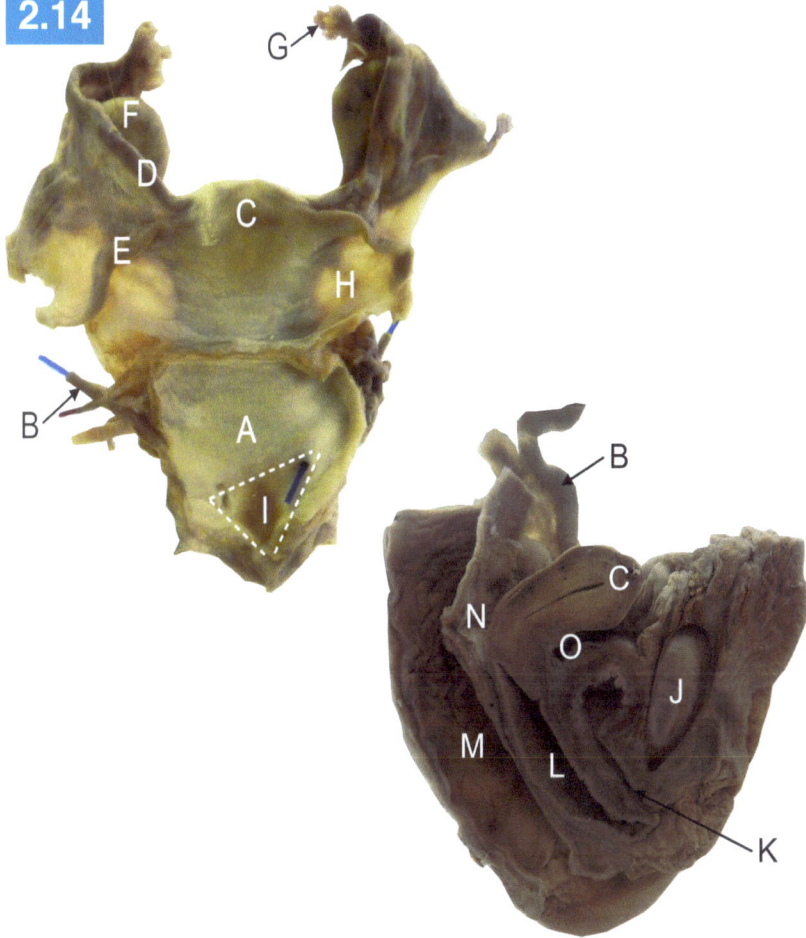

QUESTIONS

1. Label A – O.
2. Describe the position of the uterus within the pelvis.
3. Describe the relationship of the uterine artery to the ureter.
4. Where do the uterine arteries and the ovarian arteries originate?
5. To which nodes will an ovarian malignancy and a uterine malignancy spread?
6. What provides the hammock that supports the cervix?

ANSWERS

1. A – bladder; B – ureter; C – uterine fundus; D – fallopian tube; E – round ligament; F – ovary; G – fimbriae; H – broad ligament; I – trigone; J – pubic symphysis; K – urethra; L – vagina; M – rectum; N – rectouterine pouch (of Douglas); O – vesicouterine pouch.

2. The uterus lies within the true pelvis. It is angled roughly 90 degrees to the vagina and flops forwards to lie on the base of the bladder. The broad ligament is formed as the peritoneum drapes the uterus and bladder. Between the two is the vesicouterine pouch.

3. The uterine artery arises from the internal iliac artery. As the artery descends down the wall of the pelvis and approaches the uterus, the ureter descends below it, hooks around the tortuous artery and inserts in to the pelviureteric junction. This is classically taught as 'water under the bridge', where water is represented by the ureter and the uterine artery forms the bridge. In the male the bridge will be the ductus deferens.

4. Uterine arteries arise from the internal iliac arteries and the ovarian arteries, like the testicular arteries, arise from the L2 region of the abdominal aorta.

5. As lymphatics follow the blood supply, ovarian malignancies tend to spread to the aortic region, whilst uterine malignancies spread to the iliac nodes.

6. The cervical ligament provides the sacral support required to prevent uterine prolapse. The ligament acts like a hammock and has three parts to it; the pubocervical part, transverse (cardinal) cervical ligament and the uterosacral ligament. The three parts anchor the cervix to the pubic region, iliac region and sacral region respectively.

ABDOMEN

2.15

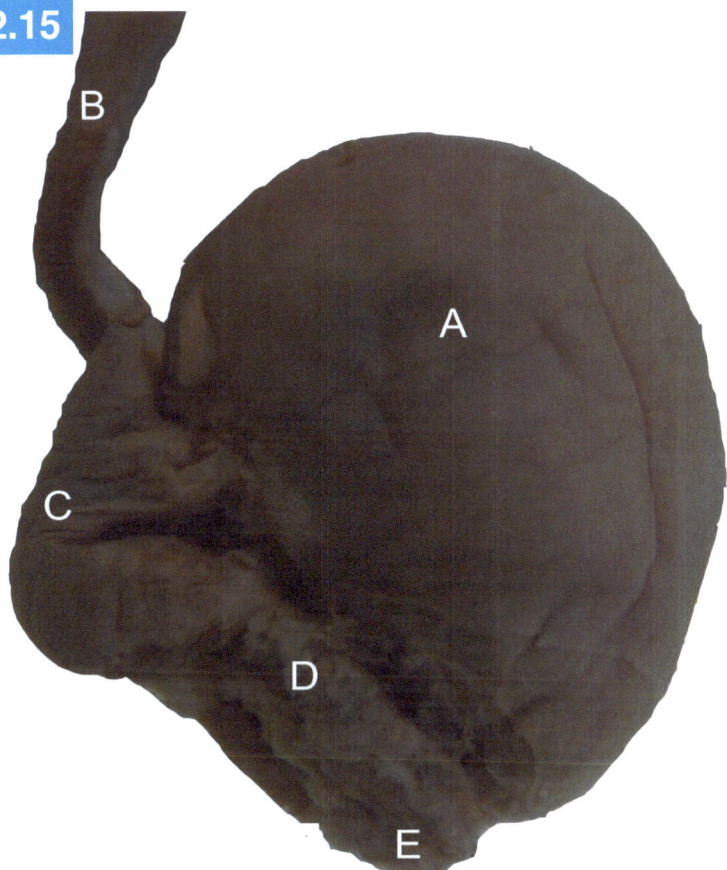

QUESTIONS

1. Name structures A – E.

2. Including the scrotum, what are the layers of tissue that cover each testis?

3. What structures are found in the spermatic cord?

4. Describe the embryological descent of the testis.

5. Describe the lymphatic drainage of the testis and scrotum

6. What are the most common types of testicular cancer?

7. What is a hydrocoele? What types do you know?

8. What is a varicocoele? What may this be a sign of?

ANSWERS

1. A – testis; B – vas deferens; C – head of epididymis; D – body of epididymis; E – tail of epididymis.

2. From superficial to deep, the layers of tissue covering each testis include: skin, superficial fascia containing dartos muscle, external spermatic fascia, cremasteric muscle, internal spermatic fascia, tunica vaginalis, tunica albuginea, testis.

3. The spermatic cord is composed of multiple structures:

3 layers of fascia	External spermatic fascia, cremasteric fascia, internal spermatic fascia
3 arteries	Testicular artery, artery to vas deferens, cremasteric artery.
3 veins	Testicular vein, pampiniform plexus of veins, vein to vas.
3 nerves	Genitofemoral nerve, sympathetic nerves, ilioinguinal nerve that runs along the outside
2 other structures	Vas deferens and lymphatic vessels

4. The gubernaculum draws the testicle from its original position on the posterior abdominal wall. Descent starts at approximately 26 weeks. At 28 weeks it reaches the inguinal canal. By weeks 28 to 40 the majority have reached the scrotum.

5. The lymph of the testes drains to the paraaortic lymph nodes. The scrotum drains to the superficial inguinal nodes.

6. Tumours of the testis can be separated into germ cell (95%) and non–germ cell tumors (5%). The majority of germ cell tumors include seminomas and teratomas. Non–germ cell tumours are primarily Leydig or Sertoli cell tumours. Testicular lymphoma is also seen in older men.

7. A hydrocele is a collection of fluid within the tunica vaginalis. A simple hydrocele involves a collection of fluid around the testis itself.
Hydrocele of the cord occurs due to segmental closure of the tunica vaginalis, causing fluid to be trapped within the spermatic cord. This may mimic an inguinal hernia. In a communicating hydrocele, failure of closure of the processus vaginalis leads to peritoneal fluid accumulating around the testis.

8. Varicocoele is a dilation and tortuosity of the pampiniform venous plexus that drains the testis. If found on the left side, it may be a sign of renal vein obstruction, potentially due to renal tumours. This is because the left gonadal vein (which drains the pampiniform plexus) drains into the left renal vein.

2.16

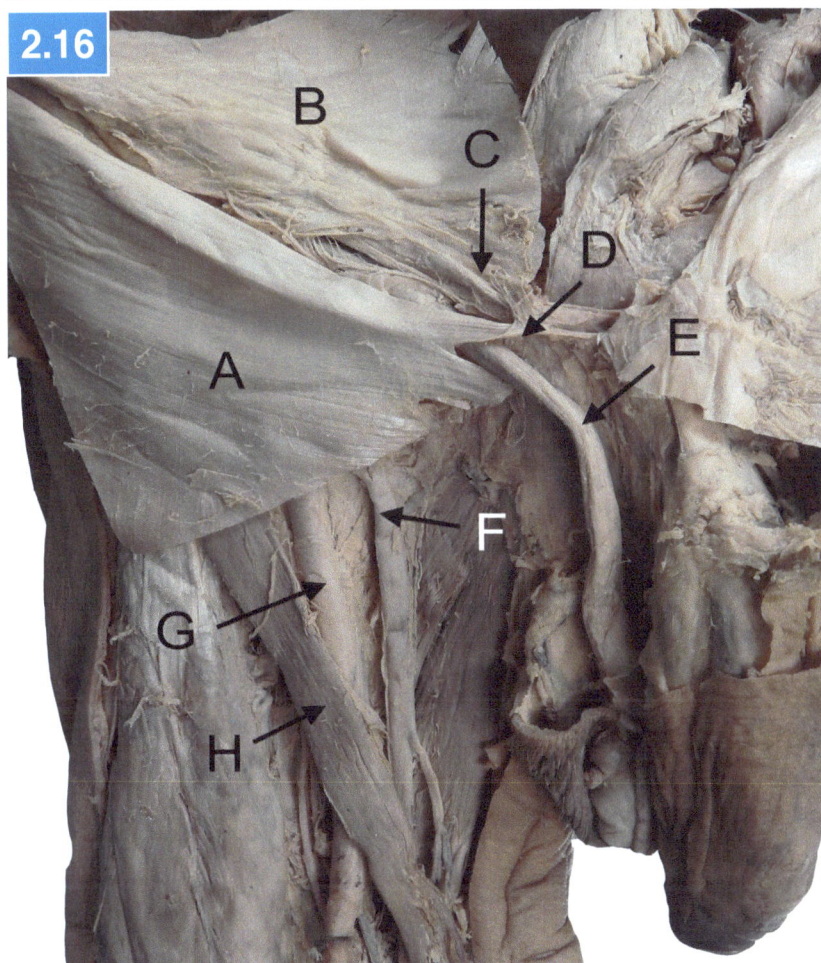

ABDOMEN

QUESTIONS

1. Identify structures A – G.

2. What are the boundaries of the inguinal canal?

3. What anatomical landmarks are used to describe the site of the deep inguinal ring?

4. Describe the approach to the inguinal canal in an open hernia repair.

5. What is Hasselbach's triangle? What is its clinical relevance?

6. What are the contents of the inguinal canal in men?

7. Where can the femoral pulse be found?

8. Name three risk factors for inguinal herniae.

ANSWERS

1. A – external oblique aponeurosis; B – internal oblique; C – conjoint tendon; D – superficial ring; E – spermatic cord; F – femoral vein; G – femoral artery; H – sartorius muscle.

2.   **Anteriorly:** Aponeurosis of external oblique. Lateral third supported by fibres of internal oblique.
Superiorly: Arching fibres of internal oblique and transversus. abdominis. The medial portion is formed by the aponeurosis of the external oblique.
Posteriorly: Transversalis fascia and the conjoint tendon medially.
Inferiorly: Inguinal ligament.

3. The deep inguinal ring is commonly described as being at the midpoint of the inguinal ligament, although the reliability of this landmark is disputed.

4. The incision made 1–2 cm above a line drawn between the pubic tubercle and the anterior superior iliac spine, from close to the midline, to about halfway along this line. Dissection is continued downwards through the subcutaneous fat and Scarpa's fascia. A vein crossing this dissection is often encountered, which should be ligated and divided. The external oblique aponeurosis is then split in the line of its fibres to enter the inguinal canal.

5. Hasselbach's or the inguinal triangle is a region of the abdominal wall. Its borders are formed by the linea semilunaris medially, the inguinal ligament inferiorly and the inferior epigastric vessels superolaterally. Direct inguinal hernias protrude through a weakened area in the transversalis fascia in this area.

6. The inguinal canal transmits the spermatic cord and ilioinguinal nerve. The spermatic cord is comprised of three layers of fascia (the external spermatic, cremasteric, internal spermatic). Three arteries (testicular, cremasteric and artery of the vas). Three veins (pampiniform plexus of veins, cremasteric vein and vein of the vas). Three nerves (nerve to the cremaster from the genitofemoral nerve, sympathetic fibres and the ilioinguinal nerve that sits on the cord). The vas deferens and lymphatics also pass within the cord.

7. The femoral pulse is found just below the mid–inguinal point, which is halfway between the pubic symphysis (not tubercle) and the anterior superior iliac spine. It is therefore just medial to the midpoint of the inguinal ligament.

8. Risk factors include: age, chronic cough/lung disease, previous herniae, obesity, pregnancy, peritoneal dialysis, constipation, connective tissue disease, male gender.

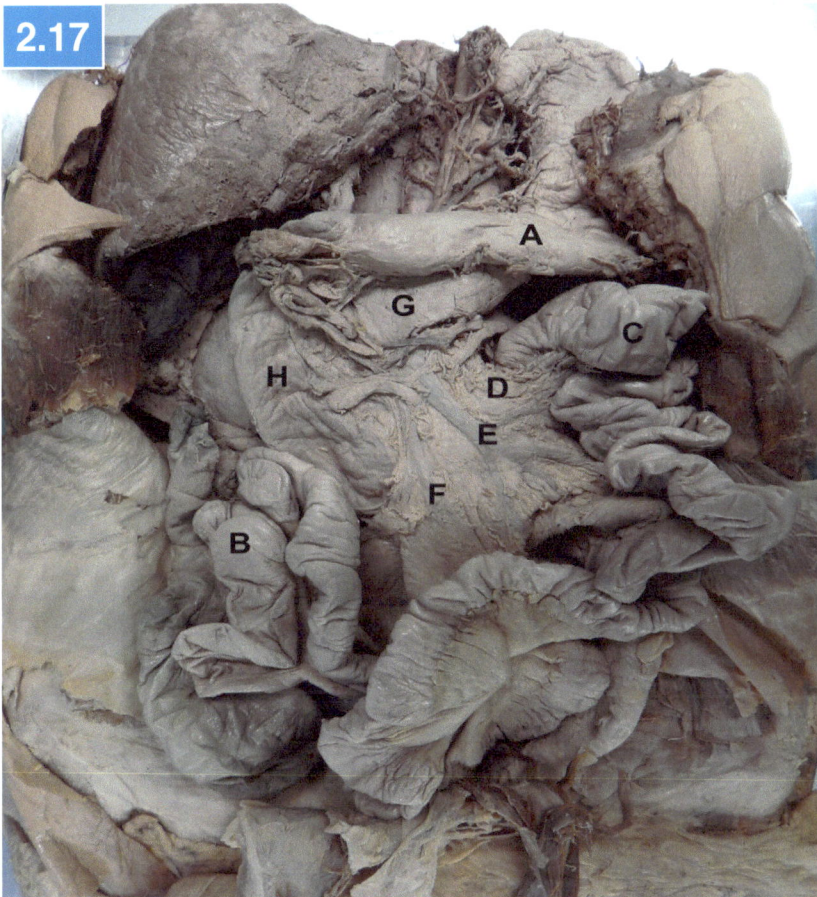

2.17

QUESTIONS

1. Name structures A – H.

2. What is the mesentery of the small bowel?

3. Where does the mesentery of the small bowel attach?

4. What is the suspensory ligament of Treitz? What is the embryological significance of this structure?

5. What parts of the bowel are intraperitoneal and which are retroperitoneal?

6. How long is a typical small bowel?

7. How may jejunum be distinguished from ileum, including the features of its mesentery?

8. What are Peyer's patches? Where may they be found?

9. What are Brunner's glands? Where may they be found?

ANSWERS

1. A – body of stomach; B – ileum; C – proximal jejunum; D – suspensory liga-ment of Treitz; E – superior mesenteric vein; F – small bowel mesentery; G – pancreas; H – duodenum.

2. The mesentery is a double layered fold of peritoneum, filled with fat, that holds the small bowel to the posterior abdominal wall and contains its supplying arteries and draining veins, as well as lymphatics and nerves.

3. The small bowel mesentery attaches in a diagonal fashion to the posterior ab-dominal wall, from the duodenojejunal (DJ) flexure to the left of the L2 vertebra, to a position overlying the upper part of the right sacroiliac joint.

4. The suspensory ligament of Treitz, also known as the suspensory muscle of the duodenum, divides the duodenum from the jejunum and the embryologi-cal foregut from the midgut. It is the place where the retroperitoneal duodenum becomes intraperitoneal jejunum.

5. The stomach, first part of duodenum, jejunum, ileum, majority of caecum, appendix, transverse colon, sigmoid and upper rectum are intraperitoneal. The remainder of the duodenum and caecum, ascending and descending colon and the middle and lower rectum are retroperitoneal.

6. The small bowel is 5 – 10 metres (15 – 32 feet) in length, averaging 7 metres (23 feet).

7. The jejunum is thicker, darker red in colour and more vascular. The mesen-teric vascular arcades are longer, with fewer arcades and its mesentery contains less fat than the ileum's. There is a gradual differentiation from one to the other.

8. Peyer's patches are aggregated lymph nodes that are found only in the ileum and thus may help distinguish this from the jejunum.

9. Brunner's glands are found only in the duodenum, proximal to the sphincter of Oddi. They produce an alkaline mucous solution to protect the intestinal walls from the acidic stomach effluent.

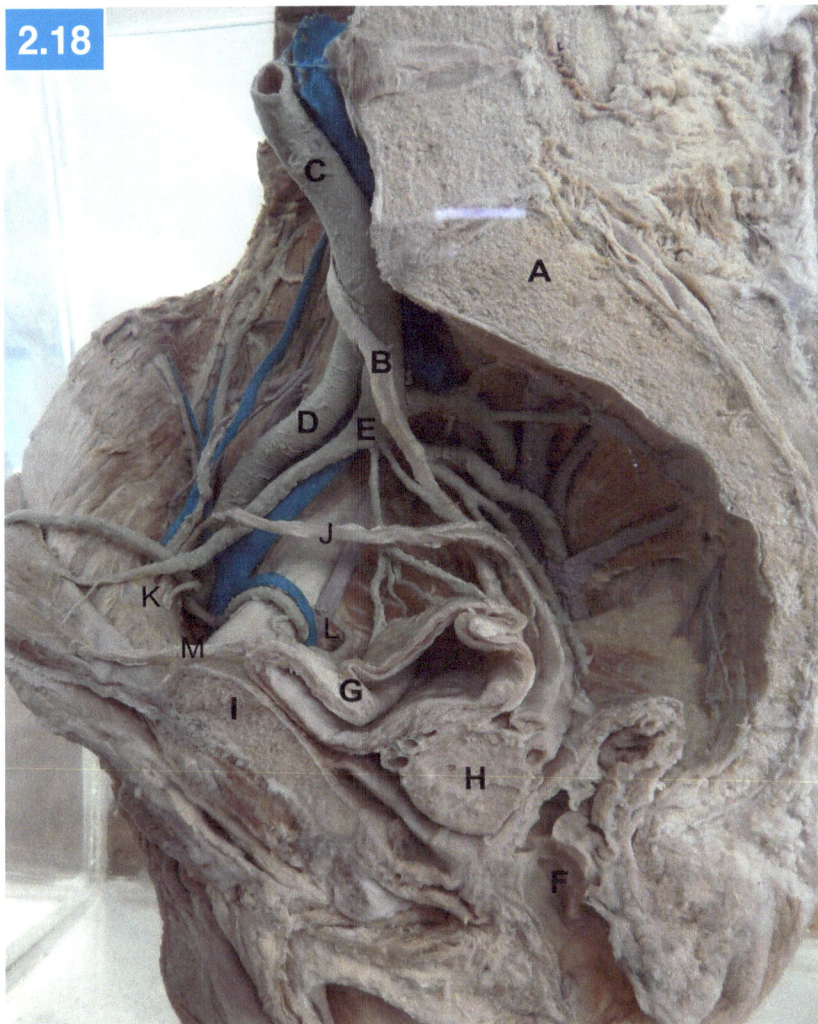

QUESTIONS

1. Name structures A – J.
2. Describe the features that confirm this is a male specimen.
3. What canal is found at K? What structures pass through here?
4. What canal is found at L? What structures pass through here?
5. What canal is found at M? What structures pass through here?
6. What are the boundaries of M?
7. What is the significance of K, L and M in clinical practice?

ANSWERS

1. A – sacrum; B – ureter; C – common iliac artery; D – external iliac artery; E – internal iliac artery; F – rectum; G – bladder; H – prostate; I – pubic symphysis; J – vas deferens.

2. The presence of the prostate below the bladder is the most obvious feature, when the external genitalia cannot be seen. Other features that can be seen here include the vas deferens, though this could be mistaken for the round ligament.

3. K is the site of the deep inguinal ring. The spermatic cord passes through.

4. L is the obturator foramen. The obturator artery, vein and nerve pass through here.

5. M is the femoral canal. It contains predominantly fat, a lymph node (of Cloquet) and efferent lymphatics.

6. The femoral canal is bordered by the inguinal ligament anteriorly, the lacunar ligament medially, the pectineal ligament posteriorly and the femoral vein laterally.

7. These are all sites of potential herniation.

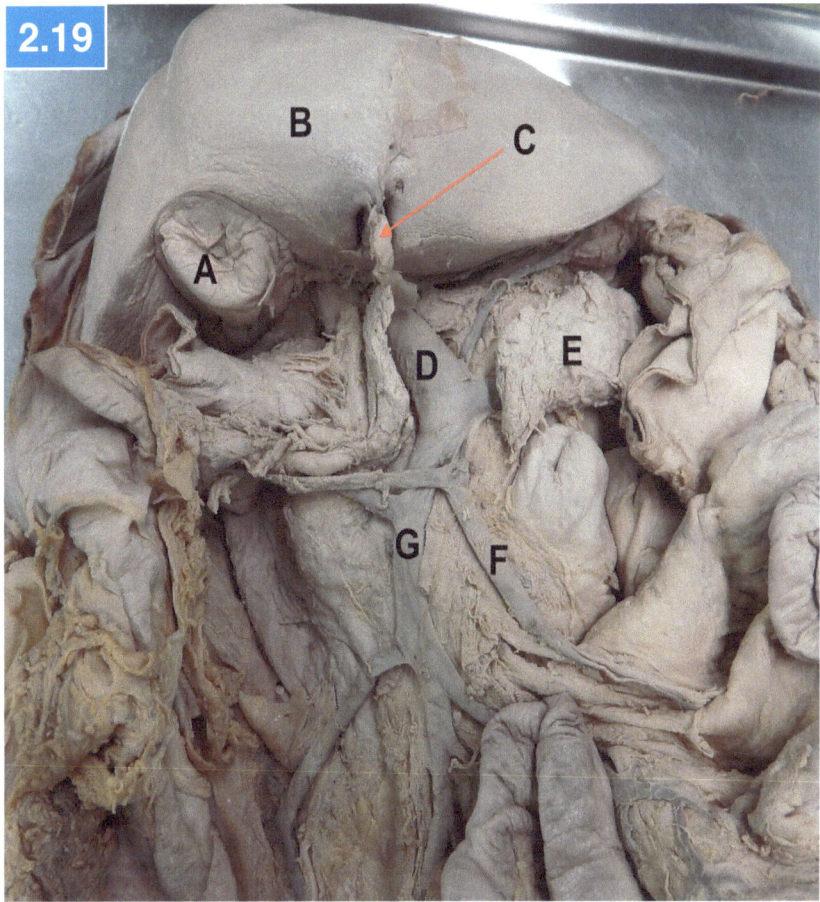

QUESTIONS

1. What is the portal circulation?
2. Name the structures labeled A – G in the above image.
3. Describe the arrangement of structures in the portal triad.
4. How many hepatic veins are there?
5. What structure from the foetal circulation is found in C?
6. What is this structure's role in the foetal circulation?
7. Into which vein does F drain?
8. Describe the numbering of the different liver segments.
9. Where may portosystemic anastomoses be found?
10. What is a TIPSS procedure?

ANSWERS

1. The portal circulation describes the venous drainage of the gut, which drains first to the liver before reaching the systemic circulation. It consists of the mesenteric and splenic veins, the union of which forms the portal vein.

2. A – gallbladder; B – right lobe of the liver; C – ligamentum teres in the falciform ligament; D – portal vein; E – pancreas; F – inferior mesenteric vein; G – superior mesenteric vein.

3. The portal vein is most posterior. The bile duct and common hepatic artery are anterior, with the artery lying medial to the duct.

4. There are three hepatic veins – right, middle and left.

5. C is the ligamentum teres, the atrophied remnant of the fetal umbilical vein

6. The umbilical vein transmits oxygenated blood from the placenta into the foetal circulation. This circulation can be very confusing – a helpful reminder is that the vein transmits blood to the fetal heart (as in life) and the umbilical arteries take blood away from the foetal heart (and onwards back to the placenta). The difference is the oxygen content of the blood.

7. The inferior mesenteric vein drains into the splenic vein.

8. Segment 1 is the caudate lobe. Segments 2 and 3 are furthest left, superior and inferior respectively, left of the falciform ligament. Segment 4 is adjacent and right of the falciform. Segments 5, 6, 7 and 8 are right of the segment 4. They are numbered in anticlockwise direction when viewed from the front, beginning with segment 5 at bottom left (the patient's left).

9. Anastomoses between the portal and systemic circulations can be found in the lower oesophagus (oesophageal branches of left gastric and azygos veins), in the abdominal wall (epigastric and paraumbilical veins), in the rectum (superior and middle/inferior rectal veins) and in the retroperitoneum. These can manifest clinically in portal hypertension, causing varices.

10. TIPSS stands for Transjugular Intrahepatic Porto–Systemic Shunt. It is an interventional radiology procedure to drain the portal vein directly into a hepatic vein, reducing resistance and hypertension in the portal system.

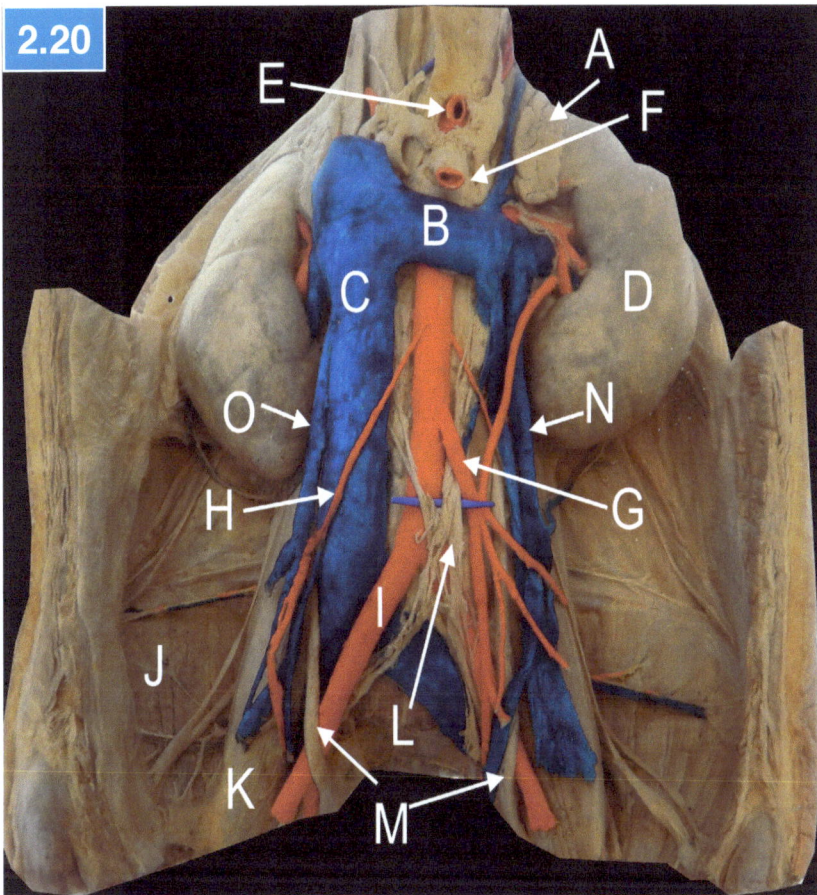

2.20

QUESTIONS

1. Name structures A – M.

2. Why does a patient with a renal stone experience colicky pain?

3. Where are the most common regions a renal stone will impact in the ureter?

4. What structure is at risk during a laparotomy incision below the level of the umbilicus?

5. Describe how the anatomy of the bladder is related to its function.

6. What structure is routinely damaged during a transurethral resection of the prostate (TURP) procedure? Why is this not detrimental?

7. Describe the blood supply to the ureters.

ANSWERS

1. A – left suprarenal gland; B – left renal vein; C – IVC; D – left kidney; E – coeliac artery; F – SMA; G – IMA; H – gonadal artery; I – common iliac artery; J – iliacus; K – psoas major; L – superior hypogastric plexus; M – ureters.

2. Colicky pain usually indicates that a hollow muscular viscus has become obstructed. The ureters are highly muscular with two layers of circular muscles and a middle longitudinal muscle.

3. Obstructions in the ureter occur when there is a transition of the lumen size from wide to narrow. The first constriction occurs at the pelvic–ureteric junction. The second area where the ureter is kinked as it passes over the common iliac vessels and descends into the true pelvis. The final site of constriction occurs at the vesico–ureteric junction (VUJ).

4. The bladder is found in the retropubic space and cannot normally be palpated. However at roughly 500 ml of urine the bladder stretches above the pubic symphysis where it can be palpated. Therefore as the surgeon approaches the suprapubic region, during a laparotomy, if no catheter has been inserted, the surgeon may enter the bladder.

5. The bladder has a smooth trigone region and a trabeculated surface. The trabeculated surface is composed of detrusor muscle arranged in a random fashion with the epithelium being made up of urothelium, which is elastic. This allows the bladder to have an enormous capacity.

6. During a transurethral resection of the prostate procedure the surgeon purposely resects the internal urethral sphincter. This contracts with sympathetic nervous system activation and relaxes with parasympathetic activation. However the master control is the external sphincter, which is innervated by somatic nerves. Therefore after this procedure the patient is still able to maintain urinary continence, though retrograde ejaculation is common.

7. The blood supply to the ureter can be divided into thirds. The upper third receives its blood supply from the renal artery, the middle from the gonadal and common iliac artery as well as the abdominal aorta. The lower third is supplied by the internal iliac artery, and all of its branches; the vesical, rectal, and in the female, the uterine and vaginal arteries.

3 | THORAX

THORAX

3.1

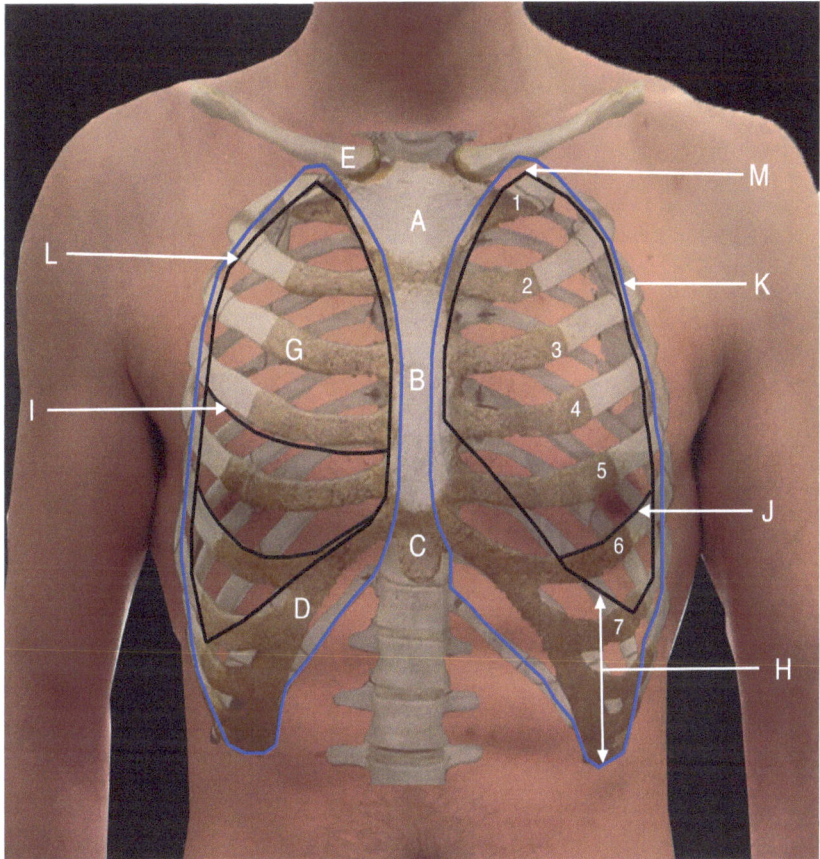

QUESTIONS

1. Name structures A – M.
2. What landmarks outline the borders of the heart?
3. Where would one auscultate for the heart valves?
4. Describe the course of each pulmonary fissure.
5. What are the surface landmarks for the parietal pleura?
6. What is the costodiaphragmatic recess?

ANSWERS

1. A – manubrium, B – sternum; C – xiphoid; D – costal margin; E – clavicle; F – scapula; G – costal cartilage; H – costodiaphragmatic recess; I – horizontal fissure; J – oblique fissure; K – parietal pleura: L – visceral pleura; M – apex.

2. The surface markings of the heart can be identified by drawing an imaginary line between these four points:
• 1 cm from the left sternal edge in the second intercostal space.
• 1 cm away from the right sternal edge in the third intercostal space.
• Fifth intercostal space, midclavicular line.
• 1 cm away from the right sternal edge in the sixth intercostal space.

3. The heart valves are best auscultated not directly over the valves but where the sounds of each valve radiate. For example, the mitral valve is not located at the apex, but that is where murmurs originating from the mitral valve are best heard. The aortic valve is best heard in the right second intercostal space and the pulmonary valve in the left second intercostal space. The mitral valve is heard in the midclavicular line in the fifth intercostal space. The tricuspid valve is best heard in the fourth intercostal space just left of the sternum.

4. The horizontal fissure can be marked on the anterior chest wall from the fourth intercostal space close to the sternum, crossing the fifth rib laterally and following the fifth intercostal space. The oblique fissure follows the medial border of the abducted scapula and arises from the third intercostal space posteriorly and descends obliquely to the sixth intercostal space anteriorly. The lower lobe is therefore heard best on the posterior chest wall.

5. The markings of the right pleura start 2.5 cm above the clavicle and descend behind the sternum. At the sixth rib it begins to change its course, descending inferolaterally towards the 8th rib in the midclavicular line, then to the tenth in the midaxillary line before finishing at the twelfth rib posteriorly. The left pleura can be marked in a similar way, taking into account its path around the heart.

6. The costodiaphragmatic recess is a potential space in the pleural cavity bounded by diaphragm and thoracic wall. The lung does not descend into this space and it is a site for fluid to accumulate, such as a pleural effusion. Anteriorly it extends from the T6 and T8 vertebral levels, in the mid axillary line it is found in between the T8 and T10 vertebrae and in the posterior chest wall it is between the T10 and T12 vertebrae.

THORAX

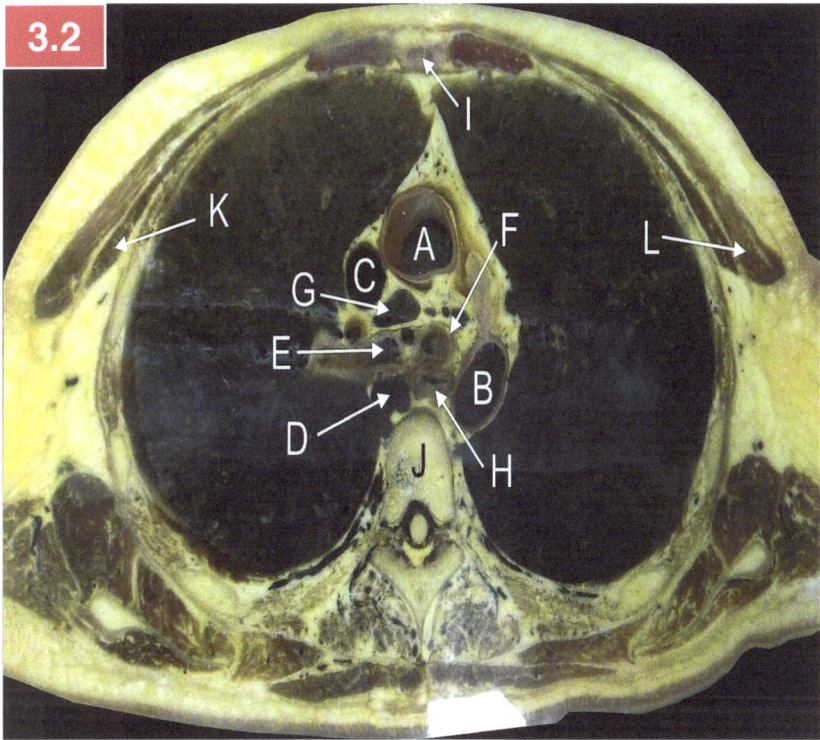

QUESTIONS

1. Name structures A – L.

2. What is the name of the plane shown in the above section?

3. What does this divide the mediastinum into?

4. Describe the course of the oesophagus.

5. At what level will the inferior vena cava enter the thorax? Where is the oesophageal hiatus found?

6. What else enters the thorax at the level of T12? What else leaves the thorax through the oesophageal hiatus?

ANSWERS

1. A – ascending aorta; B – descending aorta; C – superior vena cava; D – azygos vein; E – right main bronchus; F – left main bronchus; G –pulmonary trunk; H – oesophagus; I – cartilage of manubriosternal joint; J – T4 vertebral body; K – pectoralis minor; L – pectoralis major.

2. This is the thoracic plane, which transects through the sternal angle at the level of T4/T5. At this level will be found the carina, the azygos vein entering the SVC, the start of the aortic arch, the left recurrent laryngeal nerve and the ligamentum arteriosum.

3. The thoracic plane divides the mediastinum into the superior and inferior parts.

4. The oesophagus descends from inferior to the larynx and is a posterior mediastinal structure along most of its course. Superiorly it is found laying flat against the vertebra but at the level of T7 it becomes a more anterior relation of the descending aorta. It then leaves the thorax through the oesophageal hiatus at the level of T10. It is 25 cm long and has 5 constrictions in total, produced by the cricoid cartilage, the arch of the aorta, the left main bronchus, the left atrium and the oesophageal hiatus.

5. The inferior vena cava (IVC) is found at the level of T8 and the oesophageal hiatus is found at T10.

6. The thoracic duct enters the thorax at T12, accompanying the aorta, and the left and right vagal trunks leave at the level of T10 with the oesophagus.

3.3

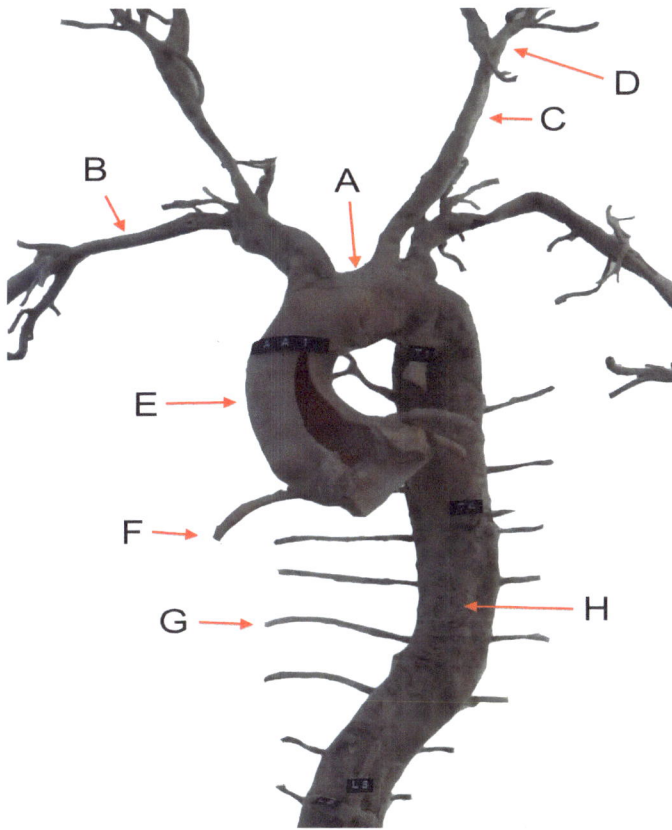

QUESTIONS

1. Name vessels A – H

2. Where does the aorta penetrate the diaphragm? What other structures pass through the diaphragm at this point?

3. At what level does the aortic arch begin and end? What are the major branches of the aortic arch?

4. The thoracic aorta has a number of branches to structures within the thoracic cavity, what do they supply?

5. Where is the ligamentum arteriosum found? What does this embryological structure represent?

6. What clinical features may be found in coarctation of the aorta?

7. Which genetic syndrome commonly features aortic coarctation?

ANSWERS

1. A – aortic arch; B – right subclavian artery; C – left common carotid; D – carotid bifurcation; E – ascending aorta; F – right coronary artery; G – posterior intercostal arteries; H – descending aorta.

2. The aorta penetrates the diaphragm at the level of T12, accompanied by the azygos vein and thoracic duct.

3. The aortic arch begins at the level of the second right sternocostal joint in the transthoracic plane (T4/5), it then arches posteriorly and to the left and becomes the descending aorta at the level of the second left sternocostal joint. It has three major branches; the brachiocephalic trunk, left common carotid and left subclavian arteries.

4. The thoracic aorta has multiple branches to structures within the thoracic cavity. In addition to the posterior intercostal arteries, there are pericardial, bronchial, oesophageal, mediastinal and phrenic branches.

5. The ligamentum arteriosum is found between the superior part of the left pulmonary artery and the proximal portion of the descending aorta. It is a remnant of the foetal ductus arteriosus. During fetal life, blood passes through here from the pulmonary to the systemic circulation, bypassing the lungs.

6. Coarctation of the aorta is a narrowing of the aorta, frequently just distal to the origin of the left subclavian artery. The clinical features vary with age. They include lightheadedness, fatigue, claudication, heart failure, upper limb hypertension and weak or absent femoral pulses.

7. Turner syndrome is the most common genetic syndrome predisposing to coarctation.

THORAX

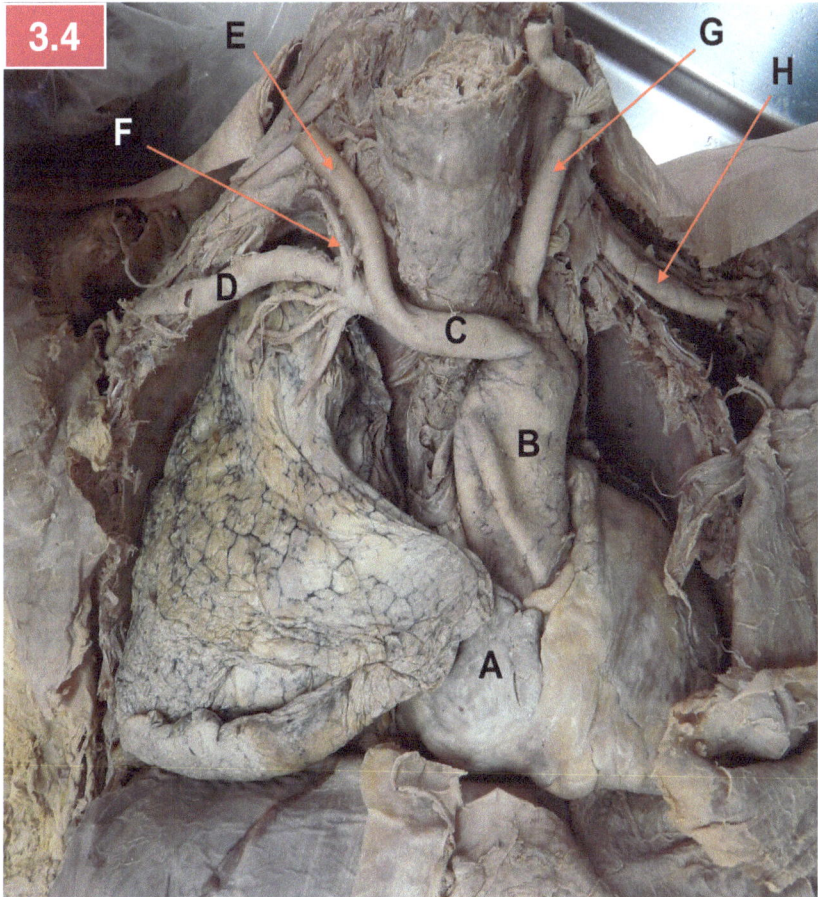

QUESTIONS

1. Name structures A – H.

2. How many parts does D have?

3. Name the branch of D that supplies the brain.

4. What does D become? What structure marks this change?

5. Are the brachiocephalic veins anterior or posterior to the great arteries?

6. What is the relationship of the subclavian artery and vein to the scalenus anterior muscle? What nerve passes anterior to this muscle?

7. What is the relationship of the vagus nerve to the main bronchi?

8. What are the first branches of B?

9. What is aortic dissection?

10. Describe a classification system for aortic dissection that you know.

ANSWERS

1. A – right atrium; B – ascending aorta; C – brachiocephalic trunk (innominate artery); D – subclavian artery; E – right common carotid; F –thyrocervical trunk; G – left common carotid artery; H – left subclavian artery.

2. D, the subclavian artery, has three parts. These are in relation the scalenus anterior muscle, behind which the artery passes.

3. The vertebral artery is the branch of the subclavian that supplies the brain.

4. The subclavian artery becomes the axillary artery at the outer margin of the first rib.

5. The brachiocephalic veins lie anterior to the arterial structures.

6. The scalenus anterior separates the subclavian artery and vein, with the artery passing posterior and the vein anterior. The phrenic nerve also passes between the artery and vein as it crosses anterior to scalenus anterior on its way to the mediastinum.

7. The vagus nerve passes posteriorly to the main bronchi; this can be a useful way of differentiating it from the phrenic nerve (which passes anterior to bronchi).

8. The first branches of the ascending aorta are the right and left coronary arteries.

9. Aortic dissection involves a tear in the tunica intima lining the artery, with pressurised blood passing between the inner two–thirds and outer third of the tunica media, creating a false lumen.

10. The Stanford system divides dissections into A (proximal aorta, with or without distal) and B (descending aorta only). The DeBakey system categorises dissections into type 1 (proximal and distal aorta), type 2 (proximal only) and type 3 (distal only). Remembering which is which may be aided by remembering that 'Stanford' has two syllables and thus two categories, where as 'DeBakey' has three.

3.5

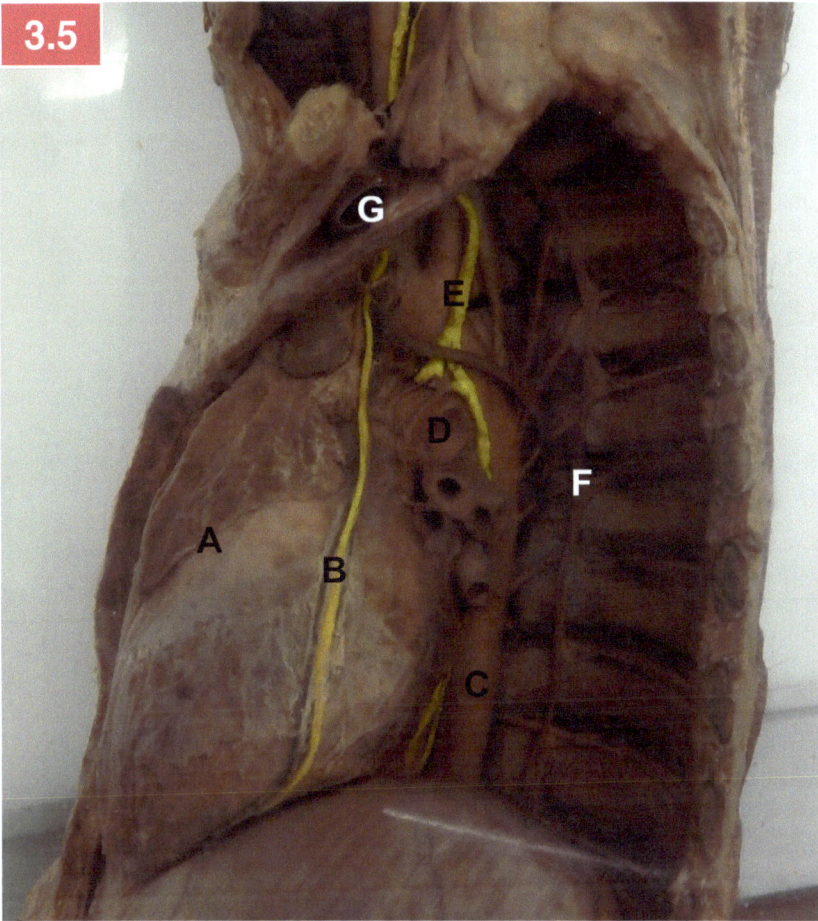

QUESTIONS

1. At what vertebral levels are the sternal angle and the xiphisternum?

2. Name structures A – G.

3. How many lobes does the right lung have?

4. At what vertebral level does the trachea bifurcate?

5. From what nerve root levels does B arise?

6. Where does E pass through the diaphragm? At which vertebral level?

7. Where does C pass through the diaphragm? At which vertebral level?

8. Describe the contents of the posterior mediastinum.

9. What are the classic features of pericardial tamponade?

ANSWERS

1. The sternal angle is at T4 and the xiphisternum at T10.

2. A – right atrioventricular groove; B –phrenic nerve; C – descending aorta; D – left main bronchus; E – vagus nerve; F – sympathetic chain; G – left subclavian artery.

3. The right lobe has three lobes – superior, middle and lower.

4. The trachea bifurcates at approximately the fifth thoracic vertebral level.

5. The phrenic nerve arises predominantly from the fourth cervical nerve root, with contributions from the third and fifth.

6. The vagus nerves pass through the diaphragm via the oesophageal hiatus, at vertebral level T10.

7. The aorta passes behind the diaphragm between the right and left crura at vertebral level T12.

8. The posterior mediastinum contains the descending aorta, the azygos and hemizygos veins, the vagus, splanchnic and sympathetic chain nerves, the oesophagus and the thoracic duct.

9. Beck's triad describes the combination of muffled heart sounds, venous distension in the neck and hypotension. The patient will classically be sat up and extremely anxious (if not yet collapsed). The triad is pathognomic for tamponade, but the full complement of signs is rarely seen.

THORAX

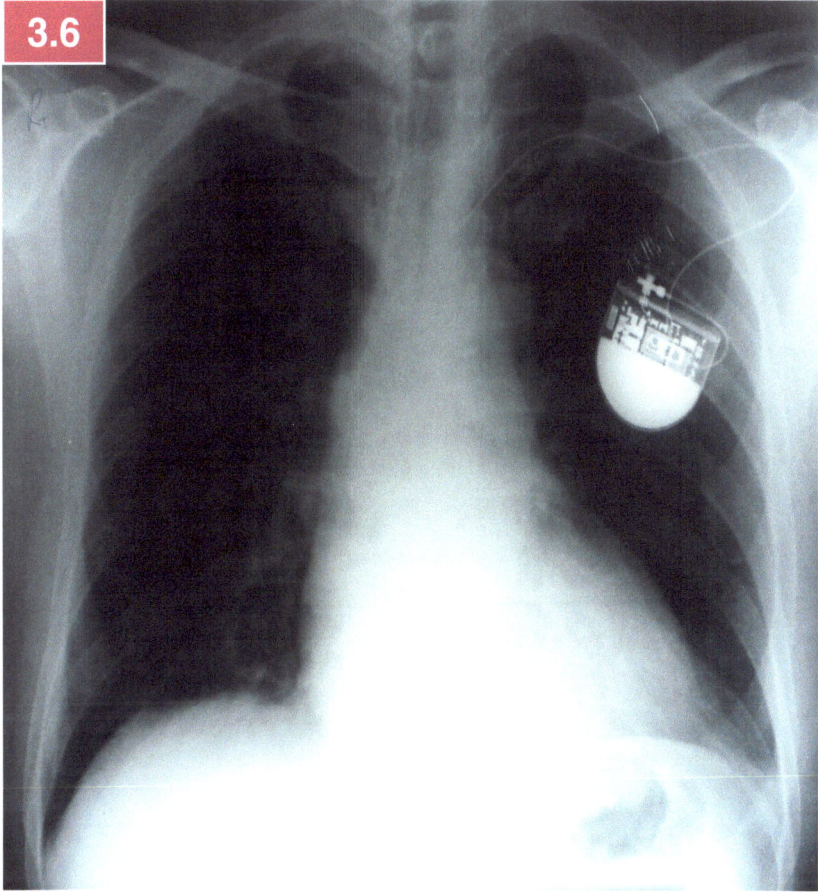

3.6

QUESTIONS

1. Describe the course of the pacing wire in this radiograph.

2. Which structures are at risk during insertion of pacemaker wires via the subclavian vein?

3. Where does the left subclavian vein originate and where does it drain?

4. Where is the body of the pacemaker placed?

5. What are the indications for permanent pacemaker insertion?

6. What is the anatomical landmark used for subclavian vein access?

ANSWERS

1. The pacing wire passes along the subclavian vein into the left brachiocephalic trunk before passing down into the superior vena cava and into the right atrium. The tip of the pacing wire is in the right ventricle.

2. The pleura may be punctured, leading to a pneumothorax or haemopneumo-thorax. The subclavian artery or brachial plexus may be injured.

3. The left subclavian vein is a continuation of the axillary vein as it passes over the first rib. It drains into the left brachiocephalic trunk, behind the left second sternocostal joint.

4. The pacemaker is most often placed in the pectoral region. This can be below the subcutaneous tissue, between the pectoralis major and minor muscles or below both pectoralis major and minor. A subcutaneous pocket is most commonly used.

5. The indications for permanent pacemaker insertion include:
- Atrioventricular block
- Sinus node dysfunction
- Intermittent bradycardia due to sinus node disease including tachy–bradycardic form.

6. The landmark for entry to the subclavian vein is inferior to the junction between the medial and middle thirds of the clavicle.

3.7

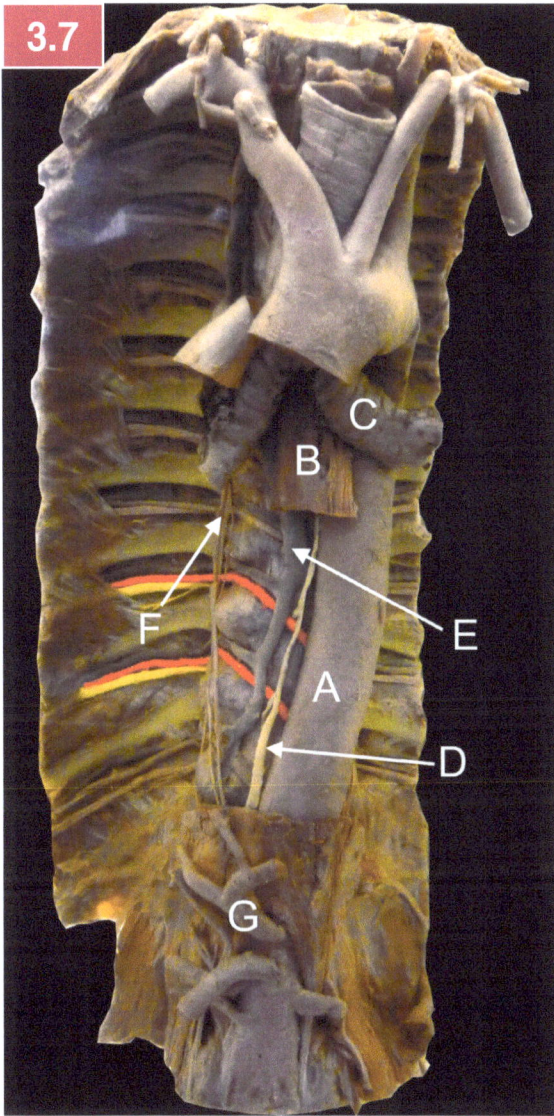

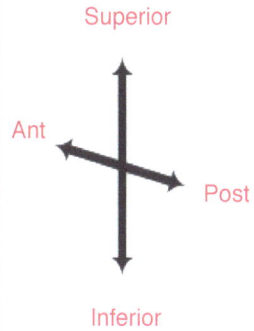

Superior

Ant ◄──────► Post

Inferior

QUESTIONS

1. Name structures A – G.

2. Describe the function of D.

3. Describe the anatomy of the sympathetic nerves.

4. Why may a patient complain of shoulder pain with a myocardial infarction?

ANSWERS

1. A – descending aorta; B – oesophagus; C – left main bronchus; D – thoracic duct; E – azygos vein; F – sympathetic chain; G – coeliac trunk.

2. The thoracic duct drains into the dilated sac of lymphatic tissue, the cisterna chyli. It circulates lymph into the angle between the left internal jugular and brachiocephalic vein. If damaged, during oesophagectomy for example, it may result in a chylothorax.

3. The sympathetic chain arises from nerve roots T1 – L2. It provides the sympathetic nervous system to the whole body. As the short preganglionic fibres leave these spinal nerves, a sympathetic chain arises along the whole length of the thoracic vertebrae, which gives off the long postganglionic fibres. This system is chiefly involved in the activation of mechanisms involved in 'fight or flight'. If the T1 root is compressed the patient may experience a Horner's syndrome.

4. The sympathetic nervous system also contributes to the cardiac plexus. The nerve roots responsible for this arise from the T1 – T5, therefore cardiac chest pain is likely to refer along these nerves, which is misinterpreted as pain arising from the T1 – T5 dermatomes (which supply the skin overlying the shoulder).

THORAX

3.8

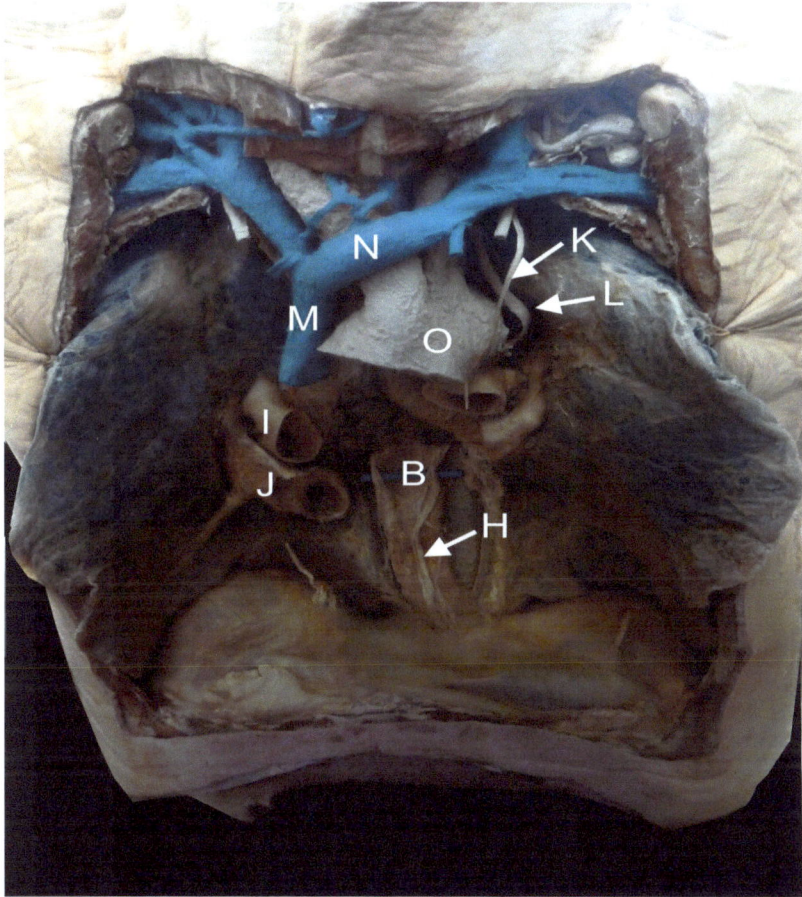

QUESTIONS

1. Name structures H – O.

2. Which vein drains the right posterior chest wall?

3. Describe the anatomy of venous flow from the left posterior chest wall.

ANSWERS

1. H – vagus nerve; I – pulmonary artery; J – pulmonary vein; K – phrenic nerve; L –vagus nerve; M – superior vena cava; N – left brachiocephalic vein; O – aortic arch.

2. The posterior chest wall veins drain into the azygos veins. This then drains into the SVC at the level of T4. The upper intercostal spaces tend to drain directly into the brachiocephalic vein.

3. The venous system draining the left posterior chest wall is slightly different. The intercostal spaces that drain spaces 3–7 enter the azygos through the accessory azygos. The hemizygos vein drains intercostal spaces 8–11.

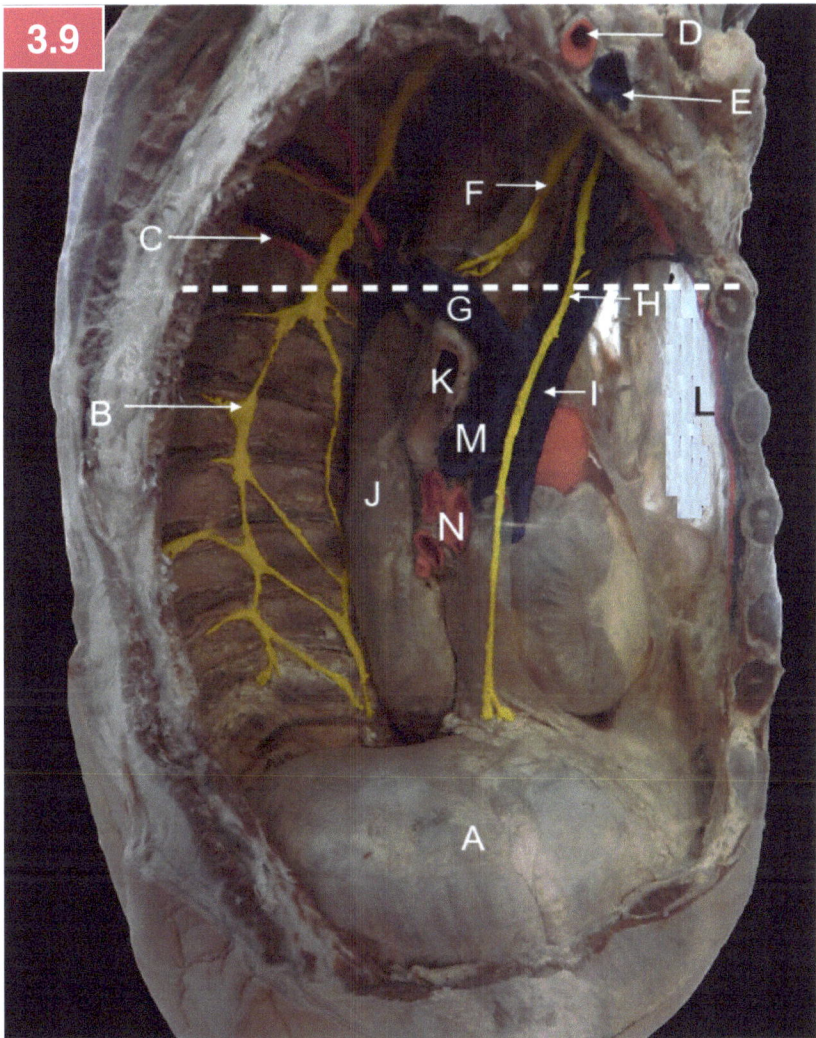

3.9

QUESTIONS

1. Name structures A – N.

2. Describe the anatomy of the mediastinum.

3. Define the transthoracic plane. What is found at this level?

4. Why may a lower–lobe pneumonia cause abdominal pain?

5. What forms the three impressions on the oesophagus within the medi-astinum?

ANSWERS

1. A – diaphragm; B – sympathetic chain; C – intercostal vessels; D – subclavian artery; E – subclavian vein; F – vagus nerve; G – azygos vein; H – phrenic nerve; I – superior vena cava; J – oesophagus; K – right main bronchus; L – sternopericardial ligament; M – pulmonary artery; N – pulmonary veins.

2. The mediastinum can be divided into four compartments. The sternal angle, (dashed line in the image overleaf) can be used to divide the mediastinum into superior and inferior. In the superior mediastinum are found the inferior vena cava, arch of the aorta, oesophagus, trachea, the phrenic and the vagus nerves. The inferior mediastinum can be divided into three compartments, anterior, middle and posterior. The anterior mediastinum is the area between the sternum and pericardium and contains a few lymph nodes, the sternopericardial ligament and the thymus. The thymus shrinks in later life and is retracted towards the superior mediastinum. The middle mediastinum contains the heart and phrenic nerves. The posterior mediastinum contains the pulmonary vessels, descending aorta, oesophagus, sympathetic chain, vertebral body, sympathetic chain, thoracic duct and the azygos–hemizygos venous system.

3. The transthoracic plane is at the level of the sternal angle and the T4/5 vertebral junction. It separates the superior and inferior mediastinum. At this level one will find the carina, the azygos vein entering the SVC, the start of the aortic arch, the left recurrent laryngeal nerve and the ligamentum arteriosum.

4. The diaphragm is mostly innervated by the phrenic nerve. The periphery is innervated by the intercostal nerves, which continue down to supply the abdominal wall. A lower–lobe pneumonia may be perceived as abdominal pain due to this pattern of innervation.

5. The oesophagus has five compressions in total but three occur in the mediastinum. The most superior is found as the aortic arch ascends over the left main bronchus and crosses the oesophagus, the second is by the left main bronchus itself and the third is the impression of the left atrium, hence the need for a transoesophageal echo to visualize the left atrium.

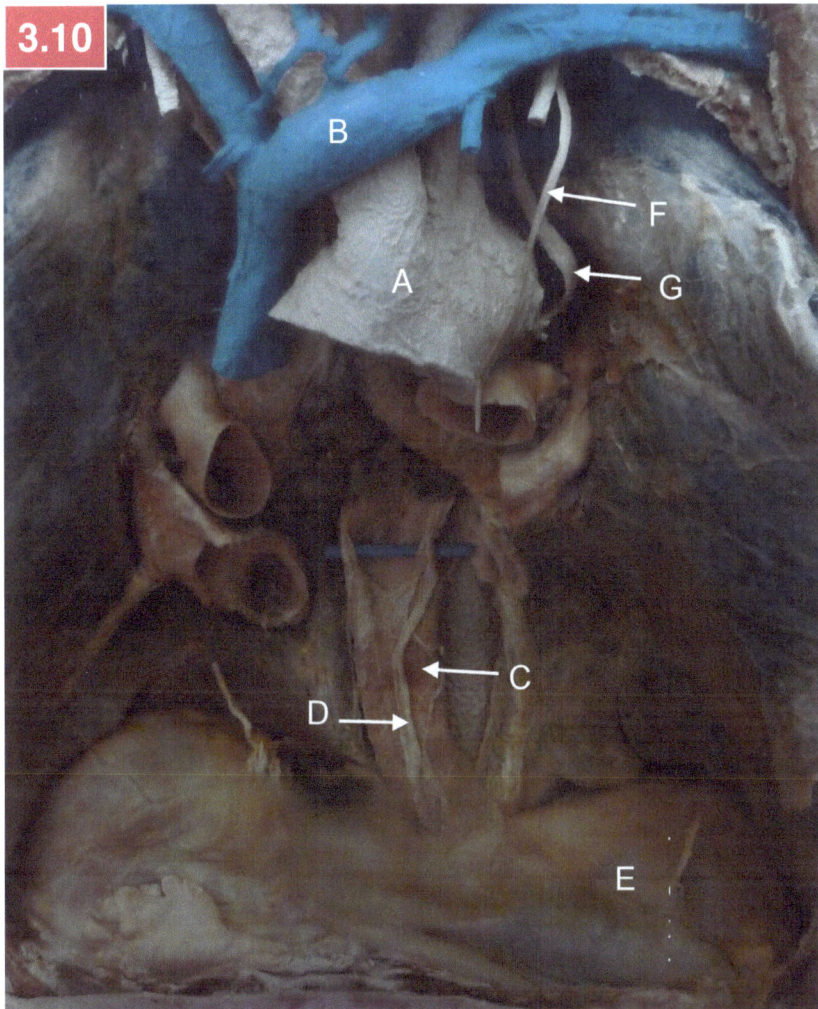

3.10

QUESTIONS

1. Identify structures A – G.

2. What structure marks the start of the oesophagus and where does it penetrate the diaphragm?

3. What are the anterior and posterior relations of the oesophagus?

4. What is the arterial supply of the oesophagus?

5. What is the Z line? What is its clinical relevance?

6. Describe the lymphatic drainage of the oesophagus.

ANSWERS

1. A – aortic arch; B – left brachiocephalic trunk; C – oesophagus;
D – left vagus nerve; E – diaphragm; F – left phrenic nerve; G – left vagus nerve

2. The oesophagus commences at the level of the cricoid cartilage at C6. It passes through the diaphragm at T10, accompanied by the vagus nerves. The right crus passes around the oesophagus. During inspiration, contraction of this region of muscle prevents reflux of gastric contents into the oesophagus.

3. Anterior to the oesophagus is the trachea proximally, the left main bronchus and left atrium. Posteriorly lie the vertebral column, thoracic duct, accessory hemizygos and hemizygos veins, and the descending aorta distally.

4. The proximal oesophagus is supplied by the inferior thyroid arteries. The middle third is supplied by branches of the bronchial arteries and direct branches from the thoracic aorta. The distal oesophagus is supplied by a branch of the left gastric artery and the left inferior phrenic artery.

5. The Z line represents the gastro–oesophageal junction. This is the site of transition from stratified squamous of the oesophagus to simple columnar epithelium of the stomach. Extension of the simple columnar epithelium into the distal oesophagus is known as Barrett's oesophagus. This is strongly associated with progression to oesophageal adenocarcinoma.

6.

Upper third	Deep cervical lymph nodes
Middle third	Posterior mediastinal nodes
Lower third	Left gastric to coeliac group of pre–aortic nodes

3.11

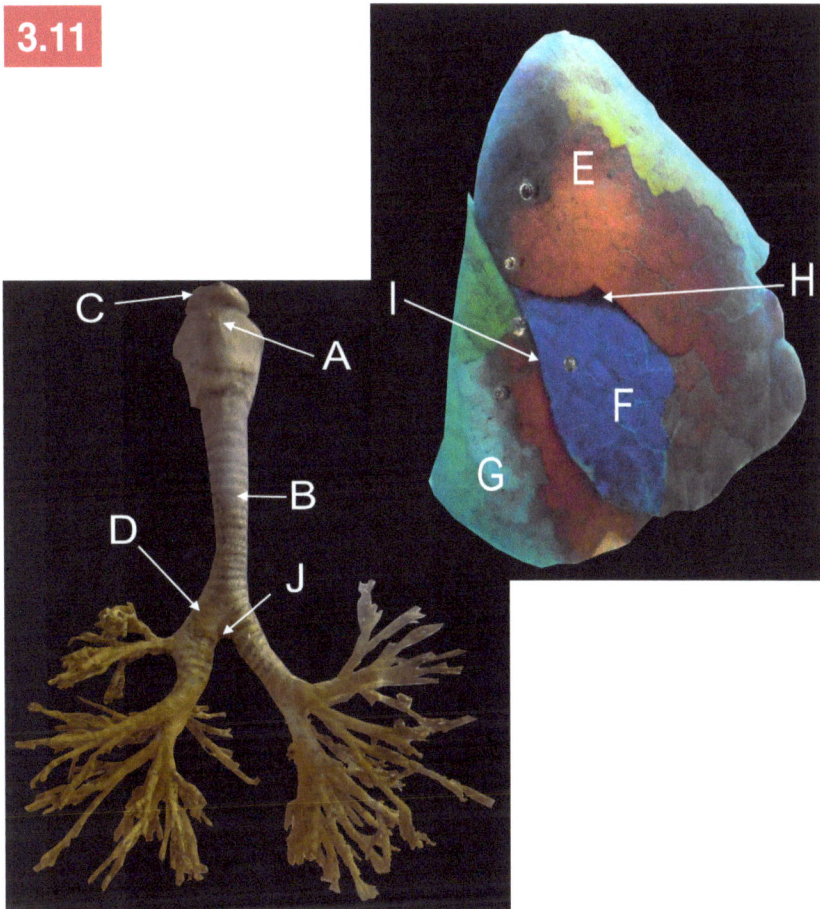

QUESTIONS

1. Label A – J.

2. Describe the structures found in the hilum of the lung and their relationships to each other.

3. How many bronchopulmonary segments lie in each lung? Why are these important?

4. Which bronchus is likely to be intubated if an endotracheal tube is inserted too far? Why is this the case?

5. Where are the best places to auscultate for the apices, upper lobe, lower lobes and middle lobe of the lung?

6. A patient with lung cancer will feel pain once which structure is breached?

7. Why is there a chance of a pneumothorax formation during central line insertion?

THORAX

ANSWERS

1. A – laryngeal prominence; B – trachea; C – cricoid cartilage; D – right main bronchus; E – upper lobe; F – middle lobe; G – lower lobe; H – horizontal fissure; I – oblique fissure; J – carina.

2. The three main structures that are involved in the formation of the hilum are the bronchi, the pulmonary arteries and the pulmonary veins. The pulmonary veins usually lie in the inferior pole of the hilum as a couplet with the artery and bronchus above it. The pulmonary artery is found anterior to the bronchus. Though the pulmonary vessels carry large volumes of blood to the lung the arterial supply to the lung parenchyma is through the bronchial arteries.

3. Each lung is divided into lobes; three on the right and two on the left. These lobes can further be classified into segments. There are 10 in each lung in total. Each segment is defined by its own blood supply and airway, allowing the thoracic surgeon to remove one segment without it affecting the other segments.

4. The right main bronchus is wider and more vertical than the left. This means that this bronchus is more likely to be intubated as well as receive inhaled foreign objects. Another characteristic is the early branching of the upper lobar bronchus from the right main bronchus.

5. The apices are best auscultated in the supraclavicular fossae. The upper lobe is best auscultated on the anterior chest wall and the lower lobe on the posterior chest wall. The middle lobe is best heard in the axilla. The upper lobes and lower lobes have confusing names as they are obliquely related, with the upper lobe as much anterior as it is superior to the lower lobe.

6. The lung is covered in visceral pleural which is tightly adherent to the lung and only has autonomic innervation. The parietal pleura is adherent to the chest wall and is innervated by the intercostal nerves. Therefore a patient will only perceive pain once the pathology involves or invades the parietal pleura.

7. Due to the obliquity of the first rib, the apices of each pleural cavity will protrude into the supraclavicular fossa roughly one inch above the first rib. This consequently leaves the apices exposed to penetration during a central line insertion.

THORAX

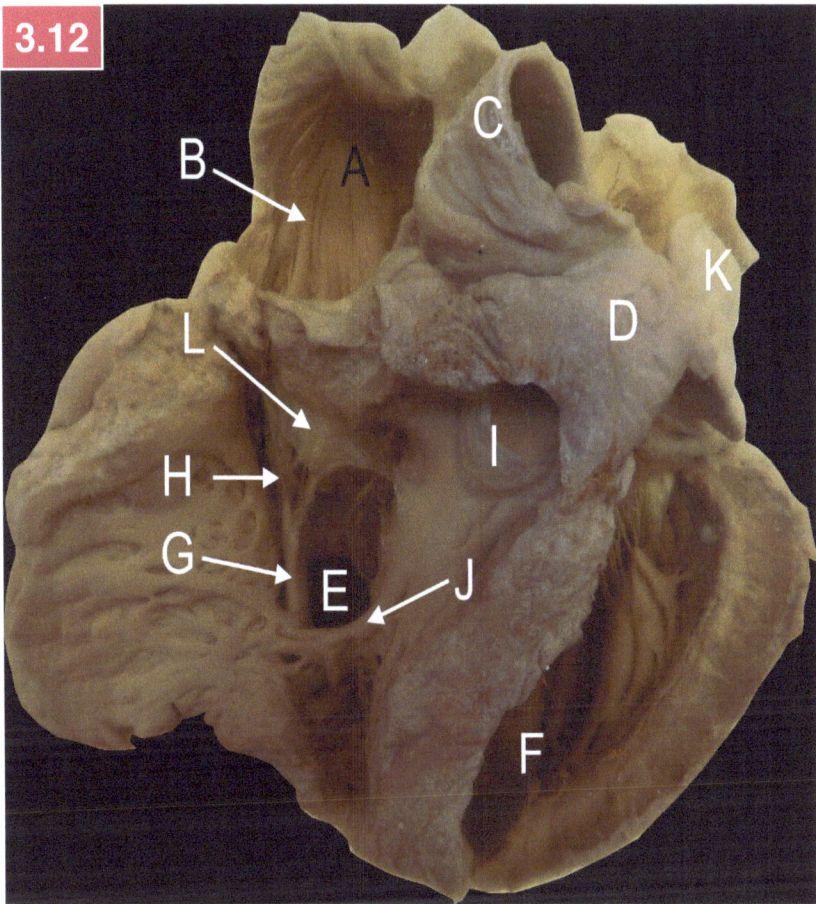

QUESTIONS

1. Name structures A – L on this anterior view of the heart.

2. Describe the orientation of the heart chambers in vivo.

3. Describe the appearance of the inner surface of the right atrium. Why does is look like this?

4. Describe the orientation of the great vessels.

5. What is the purpose of the papillary muscle?

6. What is the purpose of the foramen ovale and the ligamentum arteriosum in fetal life?

7. Describe the pathway of cardiac conduction.

ANSWERS

1. A – right atrium; B – pectinate muscle; C – aorta; D – pulmonary trunk; E – right ventricle; F – left ventricle G – papillary muscle; H – chorda tendinae; I – pulmonary valve; J – moderator band; K – left auricle, L – tricuspid valve leaflets

2. In the anatomical position the right ventricle forms most of the anterior surface of the heart with the right atrium forming the right heart border. The left ventricle contributes to the left border and the left atrium is completely posterior. Indeed the ventricles tend to lie anterior to their respective atria due to the fold-ing of the heart. Stab injuries often involve the lower pressured right chambers, though bleeding into the low volume pericardial space is quickly enough to cause cardiac tamponade, with cardiac arrest and death rapidly ensuing unless treated.

3. The right atrium has smooth and rough muscular components internally. It is mostly smooth, accounting for its low pressure. The two surfaces indicate its development from different structures. The rough muscular region indicates the primitive embryonic heart chamber surface, whereas the smooth area arises from the smooth endothelium of the blood vessels that incorporate into the atria. The crista terminalis marks the border between these two regions.

4. The aorta arises obliquely from the left ventricle and is found to the right of the pulmonary trunk. As it arches over the trunk it gives off the brachiocephalic artery, which gives rise to the right common carotid and right subclavian arter-ies. Adjacent to the brachiocephalic, the left common carotid and left subclavian arteries arise directly from the arch. The merging of the subclavian and internal jugular veins gives rise to the right and left brachiocephalic veins.

5. The papillary muscles are extensions of the trabeculated muscle of the ven-tricles, which attach to the free edge of the leaflet via the chordae tendinae. As the ventricles contract so do the papillary muscles, which will anchor and brace the leaflets of the atrioventricular valves to prevent them from prolapsing into the atria.

6. The fossa ovalis is the remnant of the foramen ovale. In utero the foramen allows the shunting of oxygenated blood, returning via the umbilical veins, to the left atrium. However the deoxygenated blood returning from the head and neck passes to the right ventricle and is forced in to the pulmonary arteries. As the collapsed lungs create a high vascular resistance within this artery, the blood is shunted through the ductus arteriosus into the arch of the aorta.

7. The heart has its own pacemaker in the roof the right atrium, the sinoatrial (SA) node. As an impulse spreads over the right atrium it reaches the atrioven-tricular (AV) node just above the tricuspid valve, which acts as a gatekeeper to allow ventricular filling prior to the right ventricle contracting. As the nerve impulse reaches the septum, it travels down the bundles of His towards the apex where the fibres split into the Purkinje fibres. The moderator band marks the fibres of the bundle of His, which innervate the papillary muscles.

THORAX

3.13

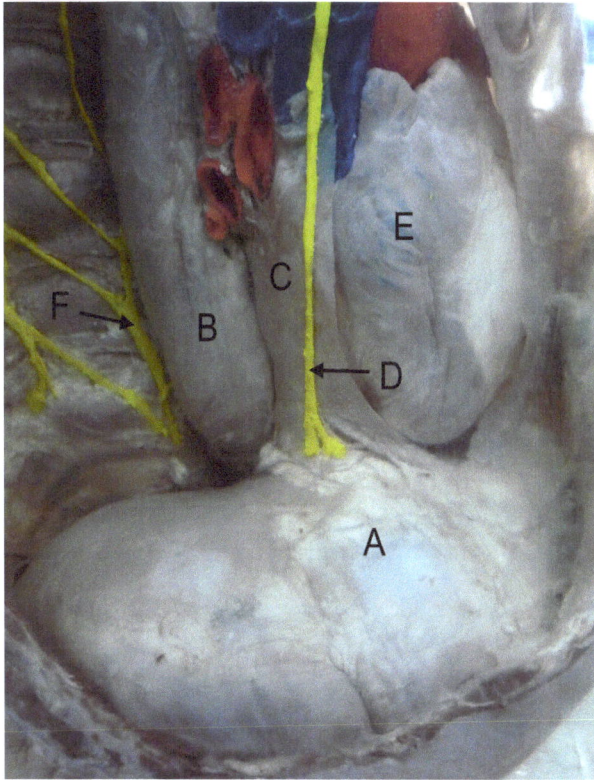

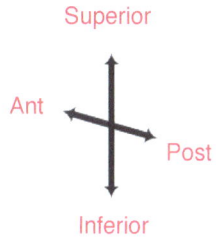

Superior

Ant

Post

Inferior

QUESTIONS

1. Name structures A – F.
2. What are the peripheral attachment sites of the diaphragm?
3. Where do the muscle fibres insert?
4. To what vertebral level do the crura of the diaphragm extend?
5. What are the three major apertures of the diaphragm? At what vertebral level are these found?
6. Describe all the structures that pass through these apertures.
7. What are the possible causes of diaphragmatic rupture?

ANSWERS

1. A – central tendon of diaphragm; B – oesophagus; C – inferior vena cava; D – right phrenic nerve; E – pericardium; F – sympathetic trunk

2. The diaphragm arises from the margins of the thoracic outlet. It extends from the xiphoid process, around the lower six costal cartilages to the two aponeurotic arches and two lumbar crura.

3. The fibres insert onto the central tendon. This thin, strong aponeurosis is situated close to the front of the thorax. The pericardium sits on its centre where it is fused to form the pericardiodiaphragmatic ligament.

4. The right crus arises from the bodies and intervertebral discs the upper three lumbar vertebrae. The left crus arises from the upper two lumbar vertebrae.

5. The major apertures include the caval opening, the oesophageal hiatus and aortic hiatus. They are found at the level of the T8, T10 and T12 respectively.

6. Multiple structures pass through these apertures. These include:
- Caval opening: inferior vena cava, terminal branches of phrenic nerve, lymphatic vessels
- Oesophageal hiatus: oesophagus, anterior and posterior branches of vagal trunks, oesophageal branches of left gastric vessels and lymphatics
- Aortic hiatus: aorta, thoracic duct, the azygos and hemizygos veins

7. This can occur due to blunt trauma, penetrating trauma or iatrogenic causes. The left hemidiaphragm is more frequently injured than the right, as the dome of the liver affords some protection.

3.14

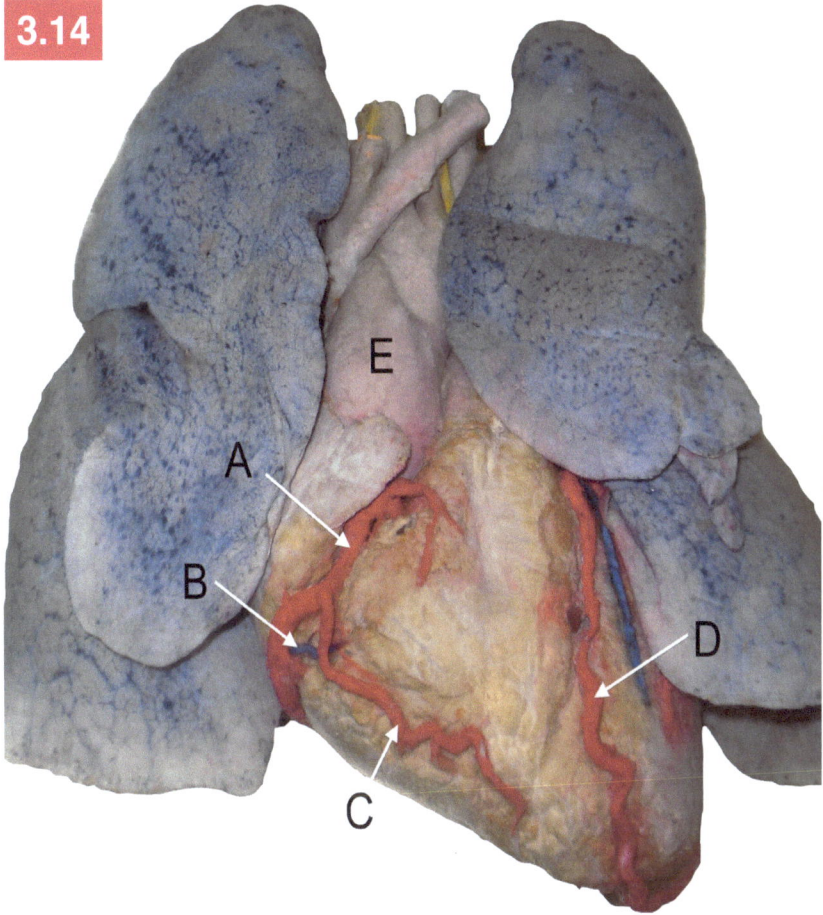

QUESTIONS

1. Name structures A – E

2. Which artery supplies the right ventricle?

3. What is meant by the term "dominance" of coronary vasculature? Which is most common?

4. Which artery supplies the sinoatrial node?

5. Where does the coronary sinus drain?

6. Occlusion of the left anterior descending artery would lead to ischaemia in which region of the myocardium?

7. Where is the great coronary vein? What is its course?

8. What features are characteristic of Tetralogy of Fallot?

ANSWERS

1. A – right coronary artery; B – anterior cardiac vein; C – marginal branch of right coronary artery; D – left anterior descending artery; E – ascending aorta.

2. The right ventricle is supplied by the right coronary artery. This originates from the anterior aortic sinus and passes along the atrioventricular sulcus.

3. Dominance refers to the vessel that supplies the posterior interventricular artery (which supplies the atrioventricular node). In 70% of people this is by the right coronary artery, in 20% it is supplied by both left and right, and in 10% the left coronary artery is the artery of origin.

4. The sinoatrial nodal artery is a branch of the right coronary artery in approximately 65% of people. In 35% it is a branch of the left coronary artery.

5. The coronary sinus drains into the right atrium. It is found in the medial wall of the right atrium between the inferior vena cava and atrioventricular valve.

6. The anterior interventricular artery is a branch of the left coronary artery. It supplies the anterolateral myocardium, including the interventricular septum, apex and a large proportion of the left ventricle.

7. The great cardiac vein passes from the apex of the heart, passes along the posterior interventricular sulcus and follows the coronary sulcus around to the left, to the back of the heart where it joins the coronary sinus.

8. Tetralogy of Fallot is a congenital heart defect characterised by the following four features:
- Pulmonary stenosis
- Ventricular septal defect
- Right ventricular hypertrophy
- Overriding aorta

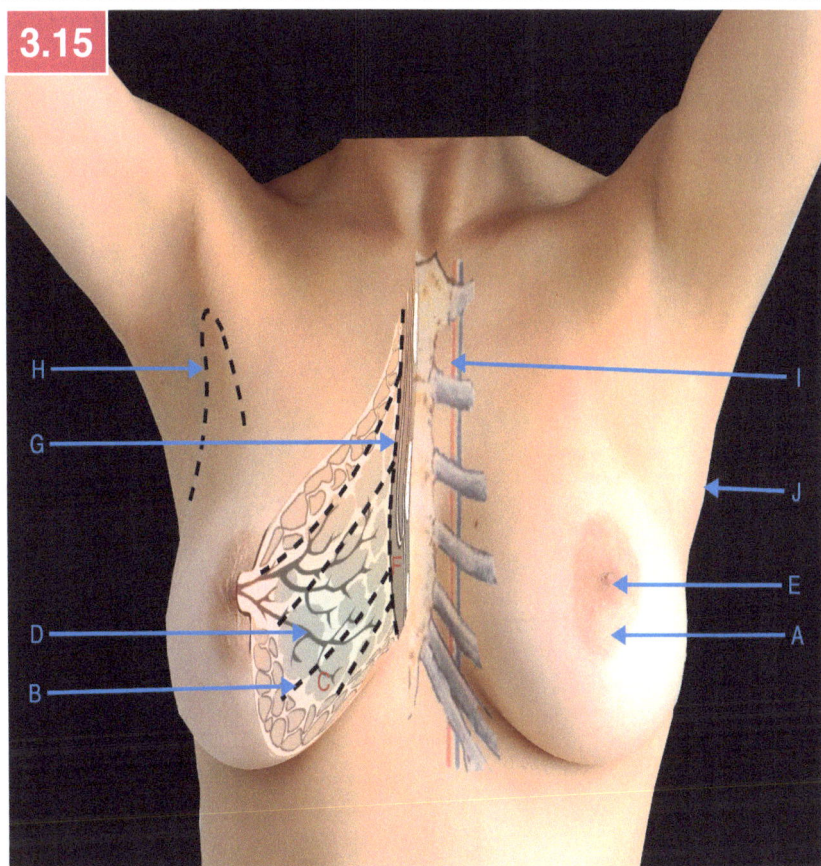

3.15

THORAX

QUESTIONS

1. Name structures A – J.

2. Describe the development of the breast.

3. Explain why nipple retraction occurs in breast cancer. What is peau d'orange?

4. To which nodes will a breast malignancy spread?

5. Why is it useful to have a woman push down on her hips during a breast examination?

6. Which nerve/s may be damaged during an axillary lymph node dissection?

7. What nerve root is responsible for nipple sensation?

8. Where is a breast cancer most commonly missed during clinical examination?

ANSWERS

1. A – areolar; B – suspensory ligament; C – lobule; D – lactiferous duct; E – nipple; F – pectoralis major; G – retromammary fascia; H – tail of Spence; I – internal thoracic artery; J – posterior axillary fold;

2. The breast is a modified sweat gland, which starts at the axilla and descends along the nipple line and comes to lie in between the 4th and 6th rib anteriorly. The nipple line extends down to the groin, which is why ectopic nipples can be found on the abdomen.

3. There are 15–20 lobules in each breast, which are compartmentalised by the suspensory ligaments (of Cooper). These ligaments arise from the retromammary fascia and insert onto the nipple. If a mass was to arise in the compartments they put tension on the ligament causing a pull and therefore retraction on the nipple. When this is coupled with subcutaneous oedema it gives a dimpling of the breast called peau d'orange (orange peel), named for its resemblance to orange peel.

4. As a general rule, lymphatic drainage follows the venous drainage to that area. There are two areas of spread; one to the axilla one to the internal thoracic nodes. Therefore a malignancy arising from the inner half of the breast may spread to the inner half of the other breast.

5. By pushing down on her hips a woman will contract her pectoralis major muscle. If a tumour is tethered to the underlying muscles the contraction will illustrate fixity to muscle.

6. The long thoracic nerve of Bell descends along the posterior axillary line and may be damaged during a lymph node clearance, resulting in winging of the scapula. The thoracodorsal nerve is also at risk; damage to this will cause loss of innervation to the latissimus dorsi. The intercostobrachial nerve crosses low through the axilla and is typically sacrificed to permit access, as it causes only minor sensory loss to the medial aspect of the upper arm

7. The T4 intercostal nerve is most commonly responsible for sensation along the distribution of the nipple line

8. Clinicians may forget to palpate along the axilla and anterior axillary line, which represents the axillary tail of Spence. This is an area where a breast malignancy may arise and can be missed if not examined thoroughly. Therefore these malignancies have a poorer prognosis as they are picked up late.

THORAX

4 | LOWER LIMB

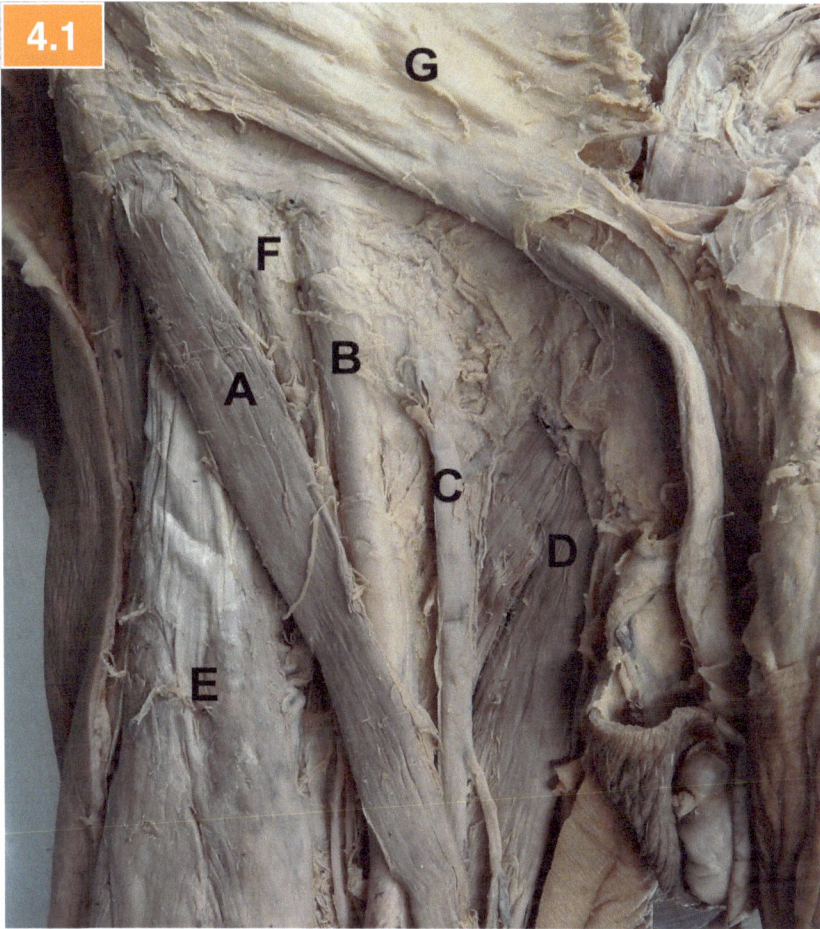

4.1

QUESTIONS

1. Identify A – G.

2. What are the borders of the femoral triangle?

3. What muscle lies in the floor of the triangle?

4. What are the surface markings of the femoral artery and the sapheno–femoral junction?

5. What are the borders of the femoral ring?

6. What is found in the femoral canal?

7. Why are post–menopausal women at greater risk of femoral herniae?

8. Why are femoral herniae usually operated on as emergencies?

9. What is the origin and insertion of E? What is its function? Which nerve innervates it?

ANSWERS

1. A – sartorius muscle; B – femoral artery; C – femoral vein; D – adductor longus; E – rectus femoris muscle; F – femoral nerve; G – external oblique aponeurosis.

2. The femoral triangle is bordered superiorly by the inguinal ligament, medially by the medial (not lateral) edge of adductor longus and laterally by the medial edge of sartorius.

3. Pectineus is found in the floor of the triangle.

4. The femoral artery is found at the mid inguinal point, which is halfway between the anterior superior iliac spine (ASIS) and the symphysis pubis. This is not to be confused with the midpoint of the inguinal ligament, which is halfway between the ASIS and the pubic tubercle, therefore slightly lateral to the mid inguinal point. This marks the site of the deep internal ring. The sapheno–femoral junction is found approximately 2–4 cm below and lateral to the pubic tubercle.

5. The femoral ring is bounded by the inguinal ligament anteriorly, the lacunar ligament medially, the pectineal ligament posteriorly and laterally by the femoral vein.

6. The single lymph node of Cloquet comprises the main content of the femoral canal. Little else is present besides fat.

7. The menopause brings a significant reduction in adipose tissue. The broader female pelvis makes the femoral ring wider and more prone to herniation in the first place; when the fatty contents is reduced there is more space for contents of the peritoneal cavity to pass through, causing a femoral hernia.

8. Despite the above, the neck of a femoral hernia is still narrow in comparison to inguinal herniae and, as such, it is at high risk of strangulation.

9. E is the rectus femoris muscle, which inserts into the quadriceps tendon, and subsequently inserts into the patella. It functions to extend the knee and can also flex the hip due to its origin at the anterior inferior iliac spine, the only quadriceps muscle that can do so. It is innervated by the femoral nerve.

4.2

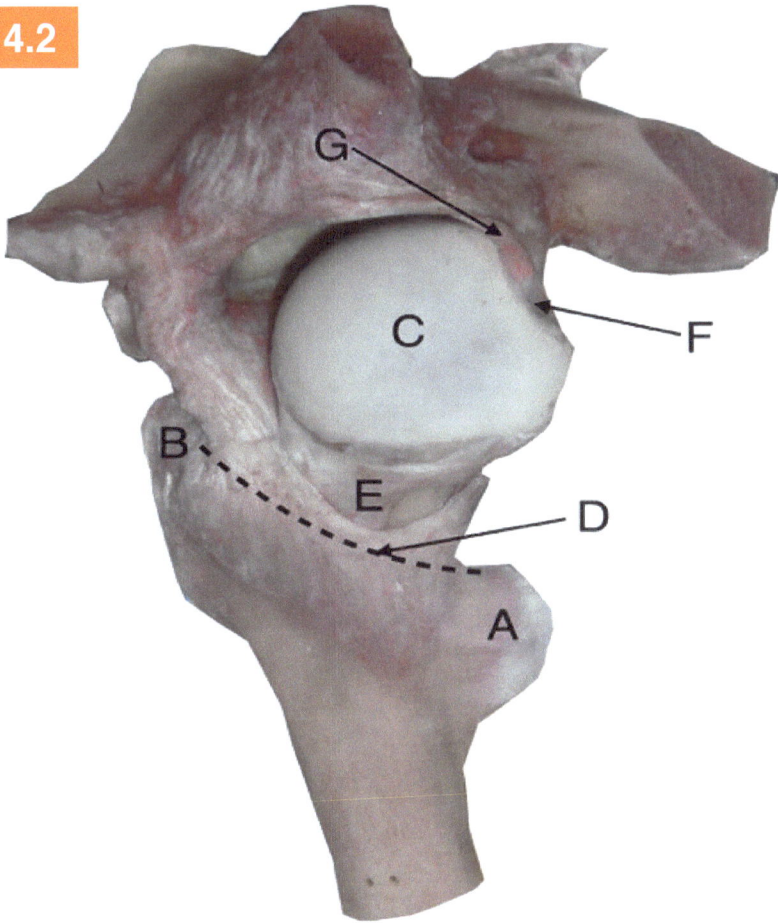

LOWER LIMB

QUESTIONS

1. Name structures A – G.

2. Describe the forces contributing to stability at the hip joint.

3. Describe the anatomy of the capsular ligaments.

4. Describe what structure lies within the ligament of the head of the femur.

5. What are the important considerations for management of an intracapsular fracture?

6. Which muscles must be reattached to the femur after performing a hip replacement?

ANSWERS

1. A – lesser trochanter; B – greater trochanter; C – femoral head; D – intertrochanteric line; E – neck of femur; F – fovea; G – ligamentum teres.

2. The hip joint is very stable and therefore requires large forces to dislocate it. Unlike the glenohumeral joint it sacrifices range of movement for stability. This is achieved by having a deep acetabular fossa, which is deepened by the acetabular labrum, to encase the whole head of femur. The joint is further reinforced by the capsule and the capsular ligaments around it. The centre of the head is also maintained within the acetabular fossa by the ligmentum teres, which attaches to the acetabular fossa.

3. The capsular ligaments include the pubofemoral, iliofemoral and ischiofemoral ligaments. The pubofemoral ligament arises from the superior ramus of the pubis and inserts into the lesser trochanter. The iliofemoral is 'Y–shaped' and arises from the ileal margin of the acetabulum and inserts into the greater and lesser trochanter. The ischiofemoral ligament arises from the ischial margin of the acetabulum to insert onto the greater trochanter. The latter is almost circular and the fibres of each ligament are like a rope, winding around one another as the hip extends, stabilising the hip further.

4. The ligament of the head of the femur (ligamentum teres) carries a branch from the obturator artery, which supplies roughly 5% of the head of femur in an adult. In childhood this artery has more of a role in development and therefore a deficiency may lead to avascular necrosis of the femoral head

5. The capsule carries nutrient arteries to the neck of femur. Disruption will lead to avascular necrosis, which commonly occurs with a displaced fracture. If significant displacement is present, orthopaedic management is invariably replacement of the femoral head and neck with a prosthesis, either as a total hip replacement in more active patients, or a hemiarthroplasty in those with lower demands.

6. It is vital to ensure any muscles that have been divided from the femur are re-attached; for example the tensor fascia lata in the lateral approach, or the deep rotators in the posterior approach. Failure to repair these structures conveys an unacceptably high risk of dislocation, and may cause an abnormal gait.

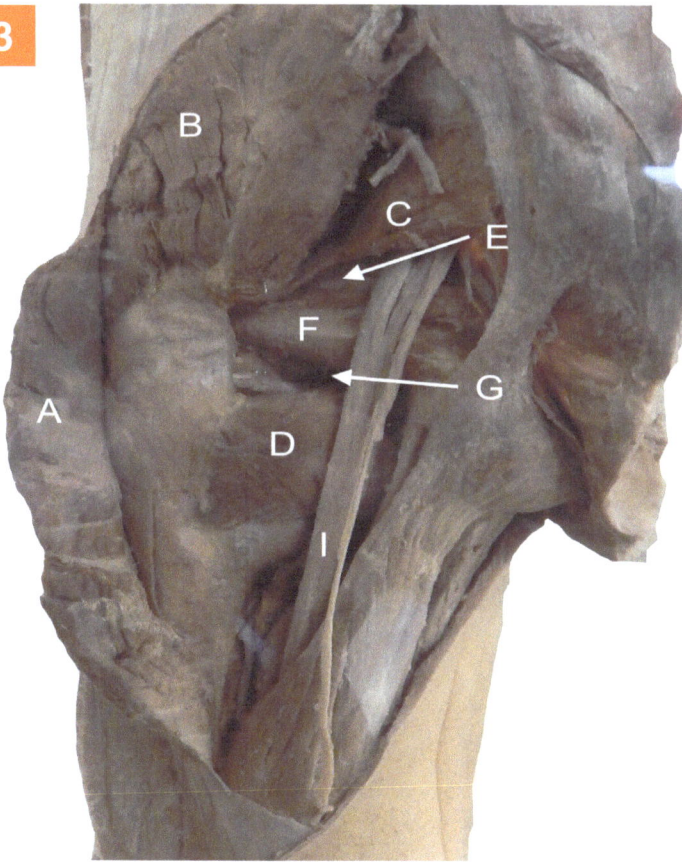

4.3

QUESTIONS

1. Identify A – B. What are their respective innervations?

2. Identify C – G. Collectively, what is their action?

3. Identify I.

4. What muscles are innervated by I in the thigh?

5. Where do these muscles originate? Identify this attachment on a specimen or the image.

6. During the posterior approach to the hip joint, D – G are divided close to the femur. What are the likely consequences if they are not repaired back to the femur?

7. Hip pain or injury may result in dysfunction of B and C. Name and describe the characteristic disability this causes.

8. The sciatic nerve leaves the pelvis through the greater sciatic foramen, most commonly under the piriformis. Name three other structures that pass through the greater sciatic foramen.

ANSWERS

1. A – gluteus maximus; B – gluteus medius. The gluteus maximus is innervated by the inferior gluteal nerve (L5, S1, S2) while the minimus and medius are innervated by the superior gluteal nerve (L4, L5, S1).

2. C – piriformis; D – quadratus femoris; E – superior gemellus; F – obturator internus; G – inferior gemellus. These are the deep external rotator group and as such, serve to externally rotate the femur. They play an important role in stabilising the femoral head in the acetabulum.

3. I – the sciatic nerve.

4. The sciatic nerve innervates the hamstring group in the thigh – biceps femoris, semimembranosus and semitendinosus.

5. The hamstrings, with the exception of the short head of biceps femoris, originate from the ischial tuberosity.

6. Failure to re–attach the deep external rotators to the greater tuberosity puts the hip at high risk of posterior dislocation post–operatively.

7. Abductor paralysis results in the Trendelenburg gait, where the upper body leans towards the affected side when that foot is planted during the stance phase of gait. Failure of the hip abductors causes the pelvis to tilt toward the contralateral side. To compensate the trunk swings towards the affected side.

This causes much confusion, but it is the upper body that 'swings' in its efforts to stabilise over the affected leg, not the lower leg 'swinging gait' seen in spastic hemiparesis.

8. Many structures pass through the greater sciatic foramen. The superior gluteal vessels and nerves pass above the piriformis muscle. Several structures pass below the piriformis including; the inferior gluteal and internal pudendal vessels, and the inferior gluteal, pudendal, sciatic, posterior femoral cutaneous nerves, nerve to obturator internus and nerve to quadratus femoris.

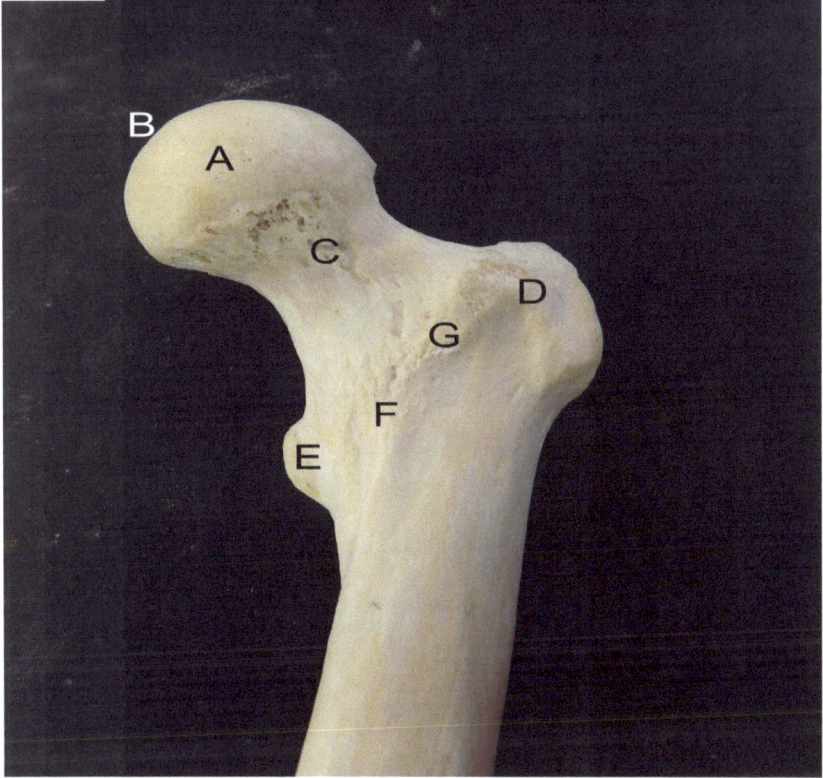

LOWER LIMB

QUESTIONS

1. Name structures A – F on this posterior view of the proximal femur. What is tubercle G?

2. Where does the capsule of the hip joint insert onto the femur? What ligaments surround the joint capsule?

3. What structures attach to the fovea?

4. Which muscle inserts onto G? What is its function?

5. Describe the blood supply to the femoral head

6. What muscles insert onto the lesser trochanter? What is their innervation and function?

7. Where do gluteus minimus and medius insert on the proximal femur? What is their function? What sign would be exhibited with dysfunction of these muscles?

8. What is the Garden classification of femoral fractures?

ANSWERS

1. A – femoral head; B – fovea; C – femoral neck; D – greater trochanter; E – lesser trochanter; F – intertrochanteric crest; G – quadrate tubercle.

2. The capsule attaches anteriorly to the intertrochanteric line of the femur. Posteriorly the capsule attaches to the neck of the femur, just proximal to the intertrochanteric crest. The iliofemoral ligament surrounds the capsule anteriorly. The pubofemoral ligament passes anteroinferiorly and the ischiofemoral ligament provides support posteroinferiorly.

3. Attached to the fovea are the round ligament of the head of the femur (previously called the ligamentum teres) and the associated artery.

4. Quadratus femoris originates on the lateral aspect of the ischium and attaches to the quadrate tubercle on the intertrochanteric crest of the proximal femur. It is part of the deep external rotator muscle group.

5. This occurs from multiple sources. An extracapsular arterial ring, formed from the medial and lateral circumflex femoral arteries, gives off perforating branches to the femoral head. A small contribution is provided by the artery of the ligament to the femoral head. In addition, the superior and inferior gluteal arteries have minor contributions.

6. Psoas major and iliacus muscles. They are powerful hip flexors. The iliacus muscle is supplied by the femoral nerve. Psoas major is innervated by anterior rami of L1–L2 with contribution from L3.

7. The gluteus minimus inserts on the anterolateral portion of the greater trochanter. The gluteus medius inserts on the lateral aspect of the greater trochanter. They are both abductors of the hip joint and are innervated by the superior gluteal nerve. Weakness of these muscles will result in a Trendelenberg gait.

8. The Garden classification is used to describe intracapsular neck of femur fractures. It has 4 stages, 1: Undisplaced incomplete. 2: Undisplaced complete. 3: Complete fracture, partially displaced. 4: Complete fracture, completely displaced.

The AO Foundation (Arbeitsgemeinschaft fur Osteosynthesefragen) provides a comprehensive femoral fracture classification system. The Garden stages are an easily memorable system for intracapsular neck of femur fractures.

4.5

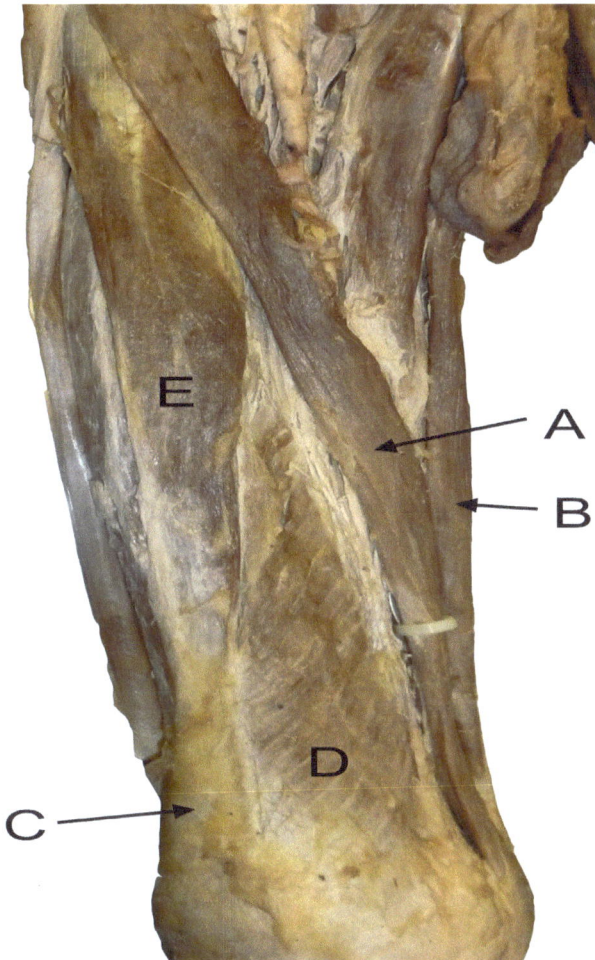

QUESTIONS

1. Name structures A – E.

2. What are the compartments of the thigh?

3. What are the origin and insertion points of muscle A? Describe its function. Which other two muscles insert in close proximity?

4. Which nerve innervates the anterior thigh?

5. What are the borders of the adductor (Hunter's) canal?

6. Describe the blood supply to the medial thigh.

7. The tendons of which muscles are most commonly harvested in anterior cruciate ligament reconstruction?

ANSWERS

1.A – sartorius; B – gracilis; C – quadriceps tendon; D – vastus medialis;
E – rectus femoris.

2. The thigh can be separated into three fascial compartments by dense connective tissue septa: medial, anterior and posterior compartments.

3. The sartorius muscle originates from the anterior superior iliac spine and inserts onto the anteromedial aspect of the upper tibia at the pes anserinus, along with the tendons of gracilis and semitendinosus. It is the longest muscle in the body. Given its broad attachment site, the sartorius muscle has multiple actions. Contraction causes flexion at both the hip and knee joints. It assists in abduction and external rotation of the thigh.

4. The femoral nerve innervates the muscles and skin of the anterior thigh.

5. The borders of the adductor canal are as follows:

Anterior:	Sartorius
Posteromedial:	Adductor longus and adductor magnus
Lateral:	Vastus medialis

The roof of the canal is formed from by the sartorius muscle and the floor by the adductor longus and magnus muscle. The lateral wall is made up of the vastus medialis muscle. The subsartorial canal should not be confused with the adductor hiatus. The hiatus is a piercing through the adductor magnus muscle at the end of the canal through which the femoral vessels and nerves pass.

6. The blood supply to the medial thigh originates from the obturator and femoral arteries. After passing through the obturator membrane, the obturator artery divides into anterior and posterior branches, which form an anastomotic ring around the obturator foramen. It supplies structures in the proximal portion of the medial thigh. The external iliac artery becomes the common femoral artery as it passes under the inguinal ligament and becomes the popliteal artery in the popliteal fossa. During its course it gives off multiple branches, the largest of which is the profunda femoris.

7. Multiple tendon grafts can be used to reconstruct the ACL ligament. These include semitendinosus, gracilis, the patella tendon, or possibly the quadriceps tendon, in addition to allografts.

4.6

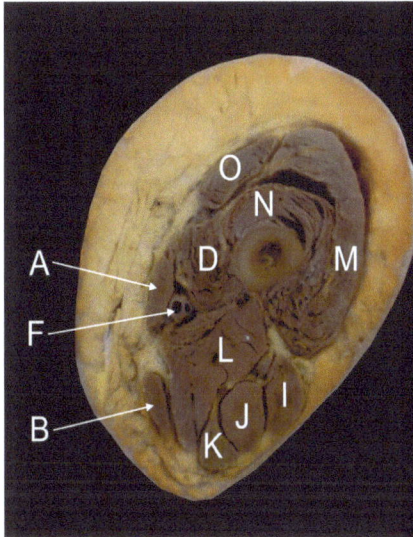

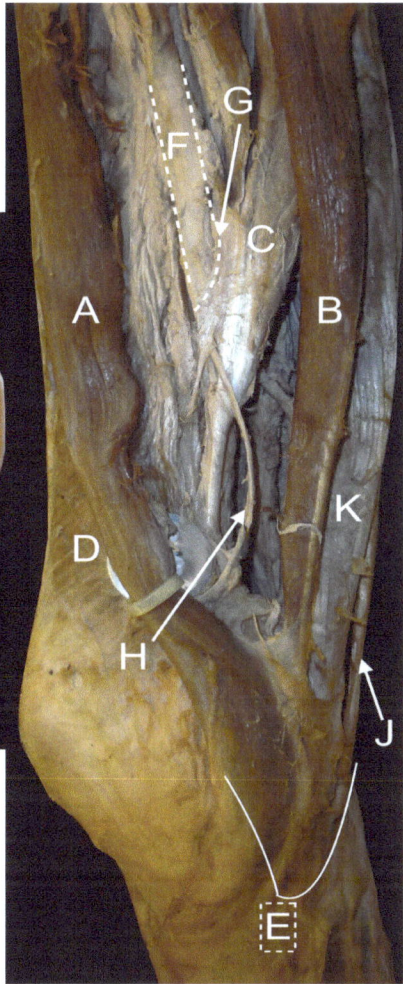

QUESTIONS

1. Name structures A – O.

2. Describe the course of the femoral artery.

3. What is the contents of the adductor canal?

4. A patient complaining of claudication within the thigh is likely to have disease where?

5. What branches arise from the profunda femoris artery?

6. What is the landmark for the adductor hiatus?

7. What is the function of the saphenous nerve?

8. Name one other nerve that enters the canal.

ANSWERS

1. A – sartorius; B – gracilis; C – adductor longus; D – vastus medialis; E – pes anserinus; F – femoral vessels; G – adductor hiatus; H – saphenous nerve; I – long head of biceps femoris; J – semitendinosus; K – semimembranosus; L – adductor magnus; M – vastus lateralis; N – vastus intermedius; O – rectus femoris.

2. The common femoral artery is the continuation of the external iliac artery below the inguinal ligament. It is found at the mid–inguinal point. The common femoral artery then gives off the profunda femoris artery and continues as the superficial femoral artery, which descends into the subsartorial canal.

3. It contains the femoral artery, femoral vein, and 2 branches of the femoral nerve: the saphenous nerve and branch to vastus medialis.

4. Claudication in a muscle is typically due to stenosis or occlusion of arteries proximal to it. Thigh claudication therefore may arise from external iliac disease, though disease further up may produce thigh as well as buttock claudication.

5. Close to its origin the profunda femoris artery gives rise to the lateral and medial circumflex arteries, which contribute to the neck of the femur. As it descends, four perforating branches are given off to the muscles and femur.

6. The landmark for the adductor hiatus lies approximately two–thirds from the ASIS to the adductor tubercle (along the course of the sartorius muscle).

7. The saphenous nerve arises from the femoral nerve and enters the adductor canal with the other vessels. It gives a branch that forms a plexus around the patella to innervate the overlying skin and descends with the greater saphenous vein to innervate the medial side of the lower leg.

8. The femoral nerve also gives off multiple branches including the nerve to the vastus medialis muscle, which also enters the subsartorial canal and innervates its corresponding muscle.

4.7

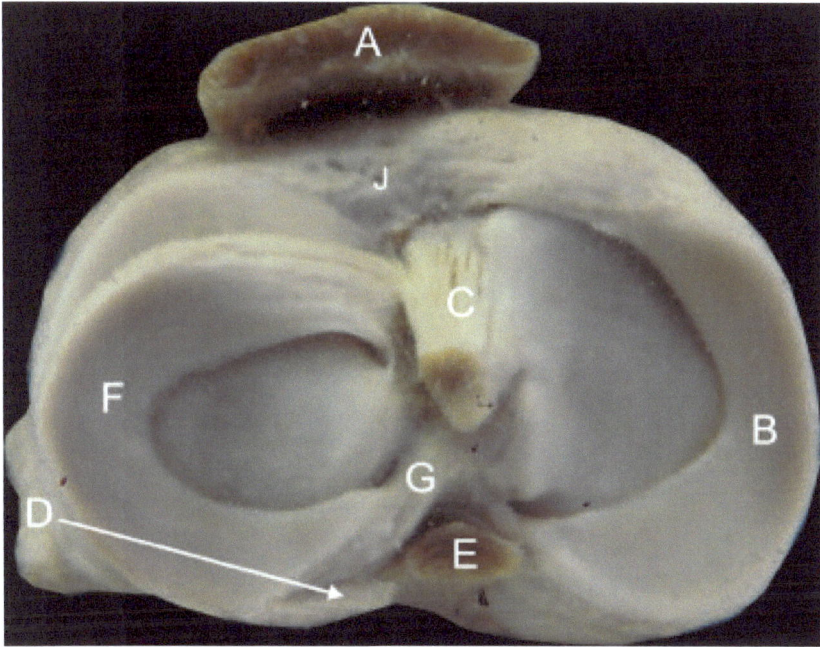

QUESTIONS

1. Name the structures A – G.

2. Inflammation of which bursa is responsible for housemaid's knee and for clergyman's knee? Where is the highest point of attachment of the capsule of the knee joint?

3. The pull of the quadriceps tendon on the patella is oblique and lateral. How is a patella dislocation prevented during extension of the leg?

4. Where can the extensor mechanism of the knee be disrupted and how could this be assessed?

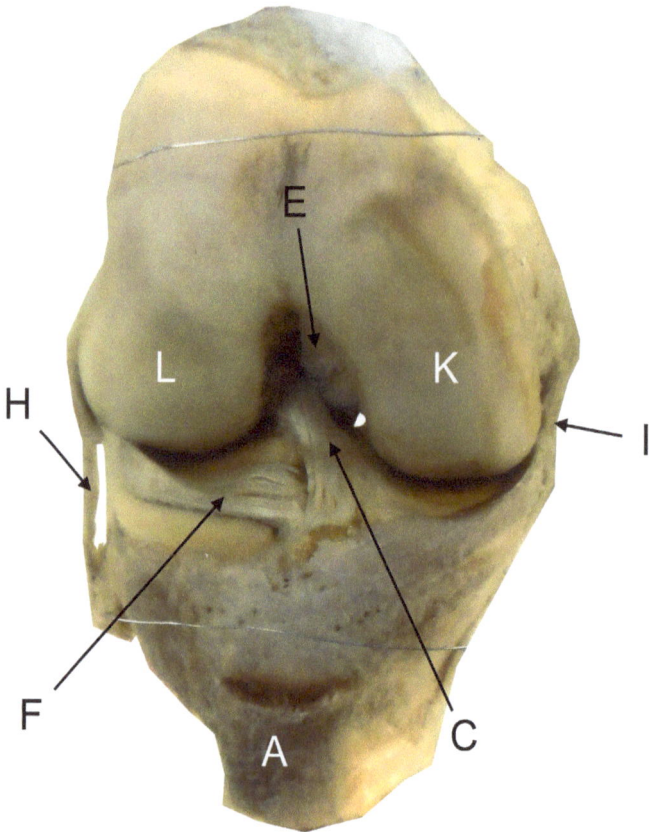

QUESTIONS

5. Name the structures H – L.

6. Describe the anatomy of the anterior and posterior cruciate ligaments.

7. How does this relate to their function?

8. What are the functions of the menisci and describe their shapes?

9. Relate the anatomy of the collateral ligaments to their function.

ANSWERS

1. A – patellar tendon; B – medial meniscus; C – anterior cruciate ligament; D – posterior meniscofemoral ligament; E – posterior cruciate ligament; F – lateral meniscus; G – anterior meniscofemoral ligament; H – lateral collateral ligament; I – medial collateral ligament; J – anterior intermeniscal ligament; K – medial condyle ; L – lateral condyle.

2. Clergyman's knee is due to an inflammation of the infrapatellar bursa and housemaid's knee is a result of prepatellar bursitis. Both are a traditionally the result of kneeling on a hard surface and differ due to the portion of the knee in contact with the floor. The suprapatellar bursa is formed by the extension of the synovial capsule, which inserts roughly one hands–breadth above the base of the patellar, on to the distal aspect of the femur. The clinical importance of this structure becomes apparent when the clinician aspirates a knee effusion.

3. The slope of the lateral articulating patellar surface of the femur is steeper than that of the medial side. This prevents the patella deviating laterally. In addition, the fibers of the vastus medialis muscle insert almost horizontally into the medial aspect of the patella. These fibers contract as the quadriceps muscle contracts pulling the patella medially, preventing it from displacing laterally.

4. Disruption of the extensor mechanism may be due to a fracture through the patella or a patellar tendon rupture. If both of these structures were damaged, this would result in a patient's inability to perform a straight leg raise.

5. ;H – lateral collateral ligament; I – medial collateral ligament; J – anterior intermeniscal ligament; K – medial condyle ; L – lateral condyle. Also: A – patellar tendon; C – anterior cruciate ligament; E – posterior cruciate ligament; F – lateral meniscus.Comapre these to the axial view of the knee on the previous page.

6. The anterior cruciate ligament arises from the medial wall of the lateral femoral condyle and gives off two bands that insert into the anteromedial (these blend with the fibers of the medial mensicus) and posterolateral aspect of the tibial plateau. If damaged, the artery within this ligament bleeds profusely and the patient will have a haemarthrosis. The posterior cruciate ligament arises from the lateral edge of the medial femoral condyle and slopes posterior and laterally to insert onto the posterior aspect of the tibial plateau.

7. As the two ligaments travel to their destinations, the fibers wind around one another like the fibers of a rope. This allows the ligaments to become tense and thus stabilise the knee. This occurs due to a slight medial rotation as the knee extends. The anterior cruciate ligament prevents displacement of the femur posteriorly on the tibia whereas the posterior cruciate ligament prevents anterior displacement of the femur on the tibia. They can be tested by the anterior draw test and posterior sag test respectively.

8. The menisci act as shock absorbers of the knee. When the knee is not weight bearing the menisci soak up the synovial fluid like a sponge and as the patient bears weight the sponges absorb the shock and the fluid is then release to keep the hyaline cartilages lubricated. The medial meniscus is more 'C' shaped compared to the smaller near–complete circle of the lateral menisci. Prior to full extension of the knee there is a slight medial rotation of the femoral condyles on the tibial plateau, known as the "screw home" mechanism. This locks the knee in full extension. Prior to the knee flexing, the popliteus muscle unlocks the knee by externally rotating the femur, allowing the knee to begin to flex.

9. The medial and lateral collateral ligaments serve to prevent valgus and varus knee deformities, respectively. The lateral collateral ligament has no attachment to the joint capsule and lateral meniscus, it is separated by a bursa. The medial collateral ligament is tightly adherent to the medical menisci and the joint cap-sule. It is likely, therefore, that damage to the medial collateral ligament will also yield damage to the medial meniscus, which in turn may damage the ACL via its attachment. This is known as the "unhappy triad".

4.8

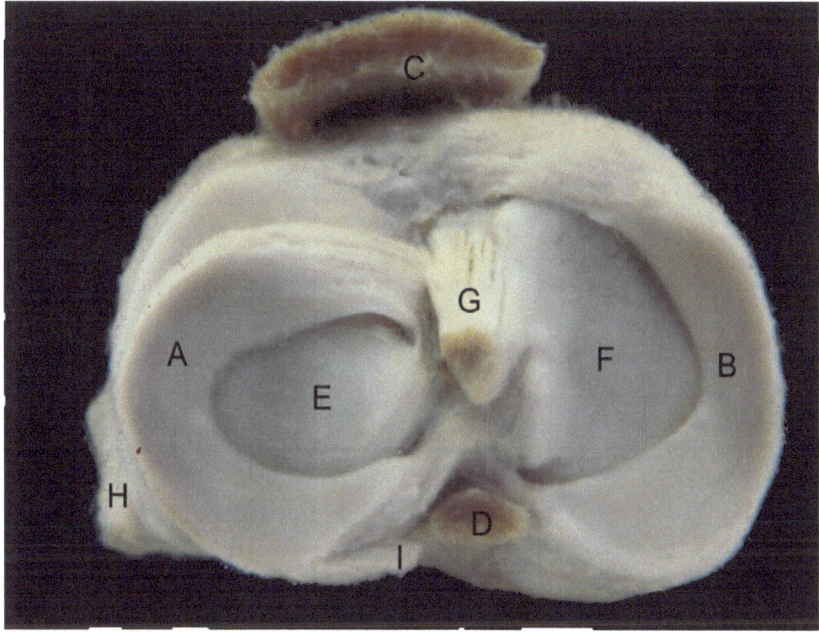

QUESTIONS

1. Name structures A – I.
2. Is this a right or left knee?
3. What are the functions of D and G? Which is the stronger?
4. Where does C attach? What is its function?
5. Describe clinical tests for the integrity of D and G. Are these accurate?
6. What are the functions of A and B? How are they classically injured?

ANSWERS

1. A – lateral meniscus; B – medial meniscus; C – patellar tendon; D – posterior cruciate ligament; E – lateral tibial plateau; F – medial tibial plateau; G – anterior cruciate ligament; H – lateral collateral ligament; I – posterior menisco–femoral ligament.

2. This is a left knee. The more "C" shaped medial meniscus is found on the right side in this image.

3. The posterior cruciate ligament prevents posterior translation of the tibial plateau on the femoral condyles. The anterior cruciate prevents anterior translation. The posterior cruciate is considered the stronger.

4. C, the patellar tendon, orginates from the inferior pole of the patella and inserts on the tibial tuberosity. Its function is as the final part of the extensor mechanism of the knee, giving an attachment to the quadriceps muscle.

5. Lachman's test can be used to assess ligamentous integrity of the anterior cruciate. The thigh is held in one examining hand and the lower leg in the other. Anterior force is applied to subject a translational force to the knee. The anterior drawer test applies this force with both examining hands to the flexed knee, with the foot anchored. Posterior cruciate integrity is assessed by examining for posterior sag or hyperextension to the relaxed knee, held aloft in extension. The posterior drawer test is similar to the anterior drawer test, but with a posteriorly directed force. As with most clinical tests in orthopaedics, these are not particularly sensitive nor specific, and are user dependent. However, they can be useful when combined with a good history.

6. The menisci serve to cushion the knee joint and distribute loading from the femoral condyles across a larger surface area of tibial plateau. They also provide some stability to the joint, particularly to torsion. They are classically injured by a twisting force to the knee – this may be accompanied by varus/valgus forces. The other ligaments are frequently injured in combination.

4.9

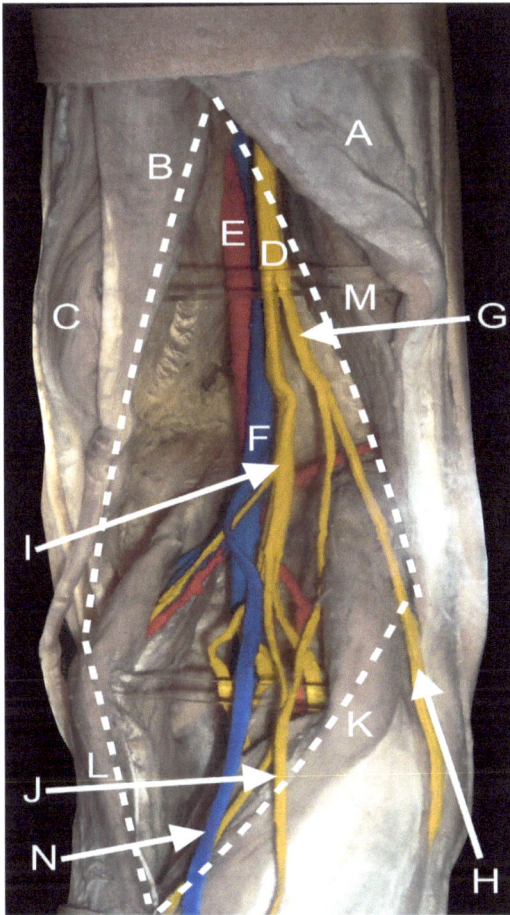

QUESTIONS

1. Name structures A – N.

2 What is the function of I?

3. What will be the likely cause of a pulsatile swelling in this area?

4. Name two other causes of a swelling in the popliteal fossa?

5. What is a Baker's cyst?

6. What is the function of J?

ANSWERS

1. A – biceps femoris (long head); B – semitendonosus; C – semimembranosus; D – sciatic nerve; E – popliteal artery; F – popliteal vein; G & H – common peroneal nerve; I – tibial nerve; J – sural nerve; K – lateral head of gastrocnemius; L – medial head of gastrocnemius; M – short head of biceps femoris; N – short saphenous vein.

2. The tibial nerve supplies the muscles in the superficial and deep posterior compartments of the lower leg, muscles of the sole of the foot, and sensation to the skin of the posterolateral lower leg and sole of the foot.

3. A pulsatile swelling in the politeal fossa would suggest an aneurysmal popliteal artery. These aneurysms are often related to chronic trauma and are said to be associated with horse riding.

4. Baker's cyst, lymphadenopathy, varicose veins, neurofibroma, lipoma. The structures of the popliteal fossa are contained by the popliteal fascia and large amounts of fat.

5. A Baker's cyst is usually found in rheumatoid arthritic patients. It as a pouch of synovial fluid that forms from the synovial lining of the knee joint, which eventually herniates through the capsule into the popliteal fossa. This usually occurs in between the medial head of gastrocnemius and the semimembranosus muscle. If ruptured, extreme pain may ensue.

6. J is the sural nerve. This nerve arises from both the tibial and common peroneal nerve and travels down the posterior aspect of the leg. Its sensory innervation is the posterior aspect of the lateral border of the foot.

4.10

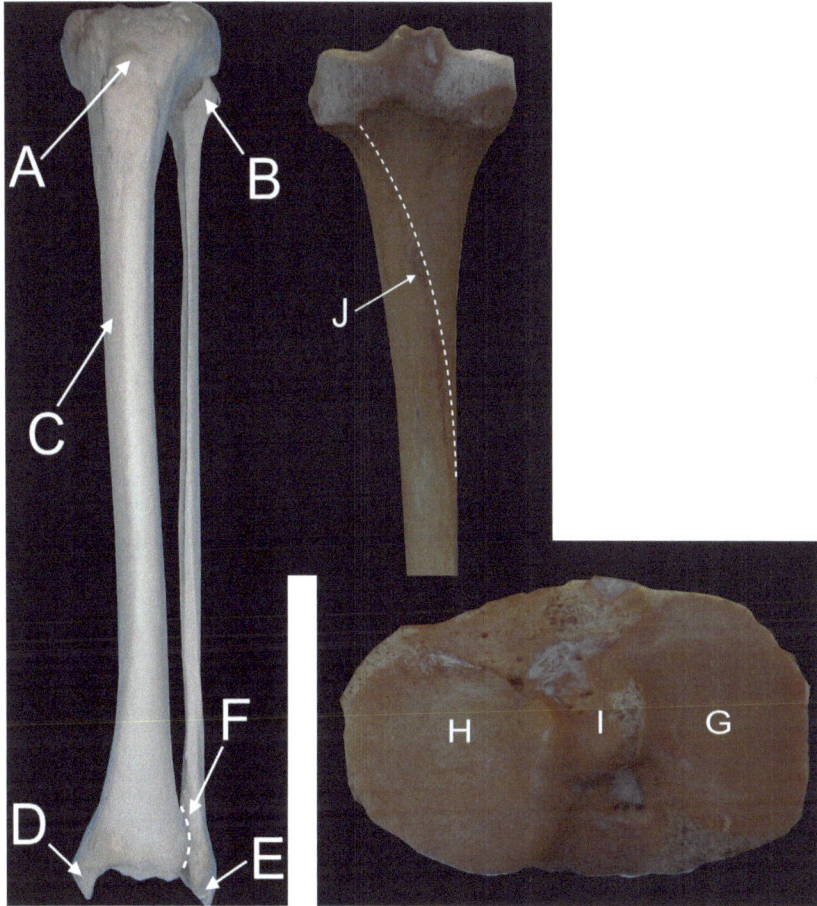

QUESTIONS

1. Name the landmarks A–J.

2. What is at risk with direct trauma at B?

3. What inserts into A? What would occur if a patient were to be struck at this point?

4. What type of joint is F? Why is it important?

5. When identifying a fracture of the tibia on an X–ray what else must one look for?

6. Name the structures that insert into the area below the medial tibial condyle, behind the medial collateral ligament.

ANSWERS

1. A – tibial tuberosity; B – fibula head; C – anteromedial surface of tibia; D – medial malleolus; E – lateral malleolus; F – syndesmosis, site of the inferior tibiofibular joint; G – medial condyle; H – lateral condyle; I – intercondylar eminence; J – soleal line.

2. The common peroneal nerve winds around the neck of the fibula and is very superficial. This can be palpated over the skin and leaves the nerve at risk of damage following trauma and it can even be damaged by application of a tight compression stockings or plaster cast. This will lead to loss of sensation over the dorsum of the foot and an inability to dorsiflex the foot, resulting in foot drop.

3. The patellar tendon inserts into the tibial tuberosity. A direct blow may lead to a rupture of the tendon leading to a high riding patella (patella alta). The patient will be unable to straight leg raise.

4. The syndesmosis is a fibrous joint. This joint is key for stability of the ankle. The Weber system of fractures classifies a fracture of the ankle below this joint (A), at the joint (B) or above the joint (C). Any disruption of this joint will lead to instability, meaning the patient will require a screw to take up the role of the syndesmosis.

5. One must carefully look and examine for fibular fractures. The tibia and fibula create a hoop, which if disrupted in one area will mean that there will be a fracture in another part of the hoop. This usually occurs due to the transmission of the force through the interosseous membrane to another part of the hoop.

6. This is where the pes anserine tendon inserts, cushioned by a bursa against the tibia, which may become inflamed. The tendon itself is composed of the conjoined tendon of the sartorius, gracilis and semitendonsus muscles.

LOWER LIMB

4.11

QUESTIONS

1. Name structures A–M.

2. What major complication may arise as a consequence of a tibial fracture?

3. Describe the anatomy of the anterior compartment of the lower leg.

4. Describe the course of the great saphenous vein.

5. Describe the innervation to each compartment.

6. Describe how you would perform a fasciotomy.

7. How will an Achilles's tendon rupture present?

ANSWERS

1. A – tibia; B – fibula; C – tibialis anterior; D – extensor digitorum longus; E peroneus longus; F – gastrocnemius; G – soleus; H – tibialis posterior; I – tendon of plantaris; J – peroneal artery; K – flexor hallucis longus; L – posterior tibial artery; M – anterior tibial artery.

2. One of the major consequences of a tibial fracture is compartment syndrome. This is a result of swelling accumulating within a closed compartment, which will compress lymphatics. This will worsen the swelling and eventually compress the veins, nerves and eventually arteries. Arterial compression is a late sign. The main symptom a patient will complain of is pain out of proportion in response to touch or movement of the muscle group within that compartment.

3. The anterior compartment contains four muscles. The tibialis anterior arises from the upper half of the tibia. Just deep to that is extensor hallucis longus. The lower half of the fibula serves the attachment of the extensor digitorum longus and peroneus tertius, which may not always be present.

4. The great saphenous vein is found on the medial side of the leg. It starts in front of the medial malleolus and is closely related with the saphenous nerve. It is at this site that cut downs are usually performed to obtain venous access. The vein passes along the medial leg to the groin, where it dives deep to join the femoral vein at the saphenofemoral junction (SFJ).

5. There are four compartments of the leg. The muscles of the superficial and deep posterior compartments receive innervation from the tibial nerve. The muscles of the anterior compartment are innervated by the deep peroneal nerve, whereas the superficial peroneal nerve innervates the muscles of the lateral compartment. The peroneal nerves arise from common peroneal nerve, which winds around the neck of the fibula. This makes the nerve prone to compression, which may present clinically as a "foot drop".

6. Two incisions would need to be made on either side of the tibia. These run along each side of the tibia, one that is 2 cm away from the medial edge and the other 2 cm from the lateral edge. These two incisions fall short of both the malleoli by roughly 5 cm. The fascia is identified and split in the line of its fibers, ensuring to open all four compartments.

7. An Achilles tendon rupture will result in an inability to plantar flex the foot. Whilst the foot is in the neutral position and the calf squeezed, the foot would normally plantar flex, though this does not occur with a tendon rupture. This is Simmond's test.

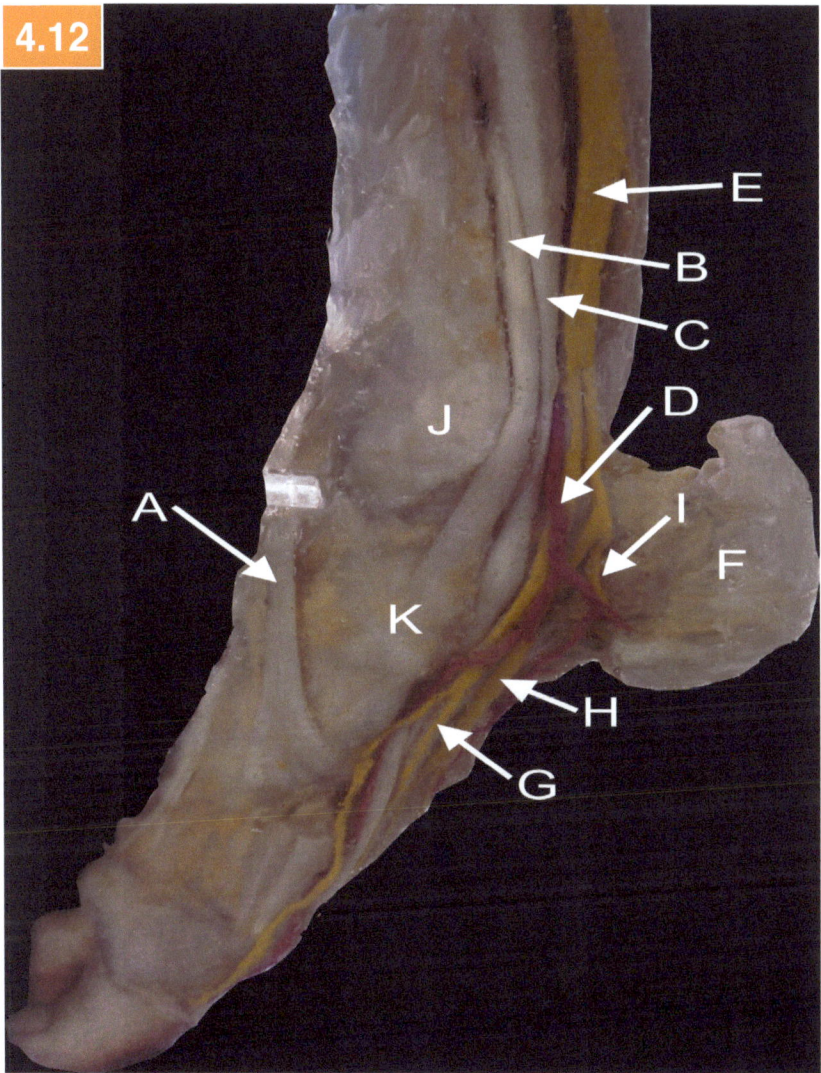

QUESTIONS

1. Name structures A – K on this medial view of the ankle.
2. What structure(s) can be palpated behind the medial malleolus?
3. Describe the anatomy of a venous cut down at the ankle.
4. Describe the stability of the medial aspect of the ankle.
5. Describe two functions of the muscles entering the tarsal tunnel

ANSWERS

1. A – tibialis anterior; B – tibialis posterior; C – flexor digitorum longus; D – tibial artery; E – tibial nerve; F – calcaneus; G – medial plantar nerve; H – lateral plantar nerve; I – calcaneal branch; J – medial malleolus; K – navicular tubercle.

2. At this landmark one may be able to palpate the posterior tibial artery. This is very important in the assessment of an ankle brachial pressure index on an arteriopath.

3. Just above the medial malleolus descend both the great saphenous vein and saphenous nerve, which supplies the skin over the medial aspect of the ankle. To perform a cut–down, a 2 cm transverse incision is made immediately in front of the medial malleolus, carefully dissecting out the vein and taking care not to damage the nerve. This is usually done in an extremis situation when other, simpler options for venous access have failed.

4. The stability of the ankle comes from the talus being housed in the mortis supported by the collateral ankle ligaments. The deltoid ligament will prevent a valgus deformity whereas the lateral ligaments will prevent a varus deformity.

5. The muscles forming the tendons that enter the tarsal tunnel have two functions. When they are all contracted they aid triceps surae (gastrocnemius and soleus) with plantar flexion and inversion of the foot. In addition to this, the flexor digitorum longus muscle will flex the 2nd to fifth toes and the flexor hallucis longus tendon will flex the great toe.

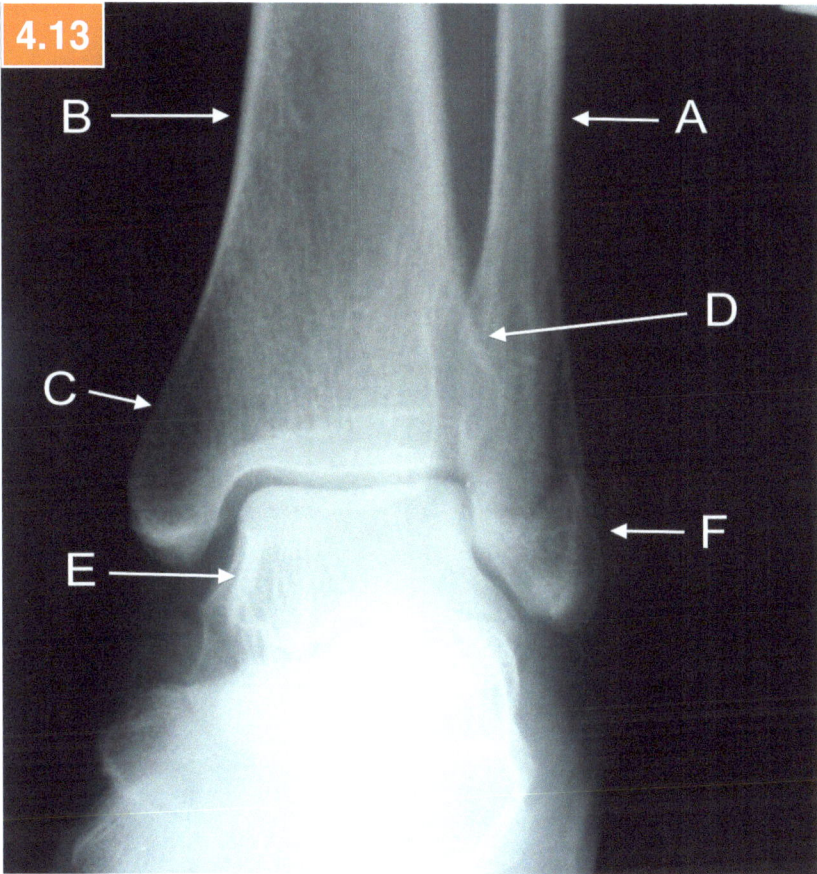

QUESTIONS

1. Label A – F.

2. Describe the bony structures that contribute to the ankle joint complex. What type of joint is this and what movements are permitted here?

3. What ligamentous structures provide support to the ankle joint complex laterally and medially?

4. What structure passes between the distal tibia and fibula and provides stability?

5. What pathology is seen on this image?

6. Describe the Weber classification of ankle fractures.

7. Avascular necrosis may occur in which proximal tarsal bone in particular?

8. The talus articulates with the calcaneus at two points. Where are these?

ANSWERS

1. A – shaft of fibula; B – shaft of tibia; C – medial malleolus; D – syndesmo-sis; E – talus; F – lateral malleolus.

2. The ankle is a synovial hinge joint that permits dorsiflexion and plantar flexion only. The proximal portion of the joint complex is formed superiorly by the distal talus, medially by the medial malleolus of the talus and laterally by the lateral malleolus of the fibula. This articulates with the talus.

3. The ankle is stabilised medially by the strong deltoid ligament. This is com-prised of four parts. The anterior and posterior tibiotalar, tibiocalcaneal and tibi-onavicular ligaments. Laterally, three individual ligaments provide support. The anterior talofibular, calcaneofibular and posterior talofibular ligaments.

4. The syndesmosis is comprised of a series of ligaments that pass between the distal tibia and fibula. They maintain the integrity of the ankle joint complex.

5. There is an oblique fracture of the lateral malleolus extending to the level of the syndesmosis, consistent with a Weber B fracture.

6. The Danis–Weber classification refers to fractures of the fibula relative to the syndesmosis.

Weber A fractures are below the level of the syndesmosis. The deltoid ligament and syndesmosis are usually intact and the ankle joint complex is stable.
Weber B fractures occur at the level of the syndesmosis. The syndesmosis is intact or partially torn. The medial malleolus may be fractured or deltoid ligament torn. There is variable stability.
Weber C fractures occur above the level of the syndemosis. This leads to disruption of the syndesmosis with medial malleolus fracture or deltoid ligament injury. The ankle complex is unstable.

7. The body of the talus is at risk of avascular necrosis. It is supplied by multiple small vessels. A large portion of the talus is covered by articular cartilage, which is not penetrated by these vessels.

8. The talocalcaneal joint is comprised of two separate articulations each with its own synovial cavity. The anterior talocalcaneal articulation occurs between the two facets on the anterior aspect of the calcaneus, including the sustentaculum tali and two corresponding facets on the inferior surface of the talus. The pos-terior talocalcaneal articulation occurs between a convex surface on the middle third of the calcaneus and a concave area on the body of the talus.

4.14

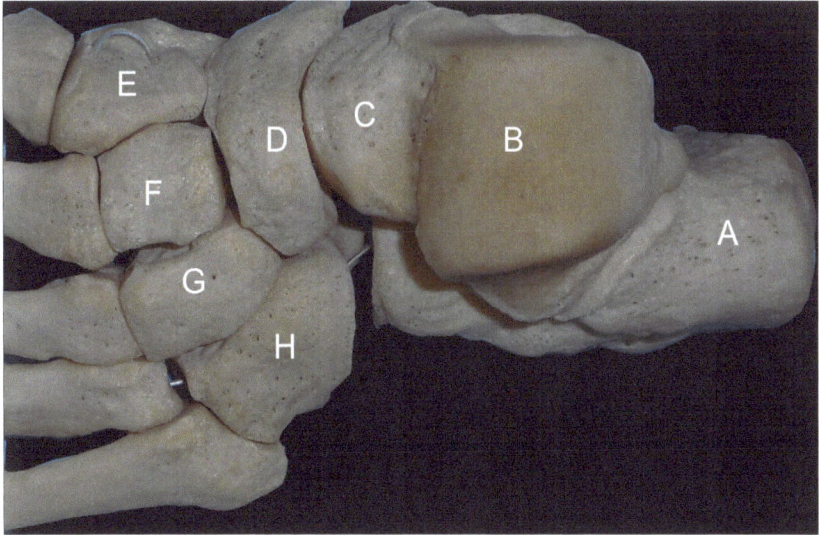

QUESTIONS

1. Name structures A – H.
2. Describe how the talus articulates with the midfoot bones.
3. What is the importance of the subtalar joint?
4. Describe the course of the peroneus longus tendon.
5. What type of fracture will occur at its insertion?

ANSWERS

1. A – calcaneus; B – talus; C – head of the talus; D – navicular; E – medial cuneiform; F – intermediate cuneiform; G – lateral cuneiform; H – cuboid.

2. The head of the talus articulates with both the navicular and the calcaneum as it sits on the shelf of the calcaneus (sustentaculum tali). The navicular and calcaneum together form a socket that is deficient on its inferior aspect but completed by a ligament, the calcaneonavicular ligament (spring ligament). These three bones and a ligament form a ball and socket joint.

3. The subtalar joint is a condylar joint that works with the mortis hinge to allow inversion and eversion of the ankle while in plantar flexion and dorsiflexion respectively.

4. The peroneus longus muscle descends along the lateral aspect of the fibula and runs underneath the foot obliquely towards the head of the first metatarsal, where it inserts.

5. A fracture at this point is associated with a dislocation and is termed a Lisfranc fracture.

4.15

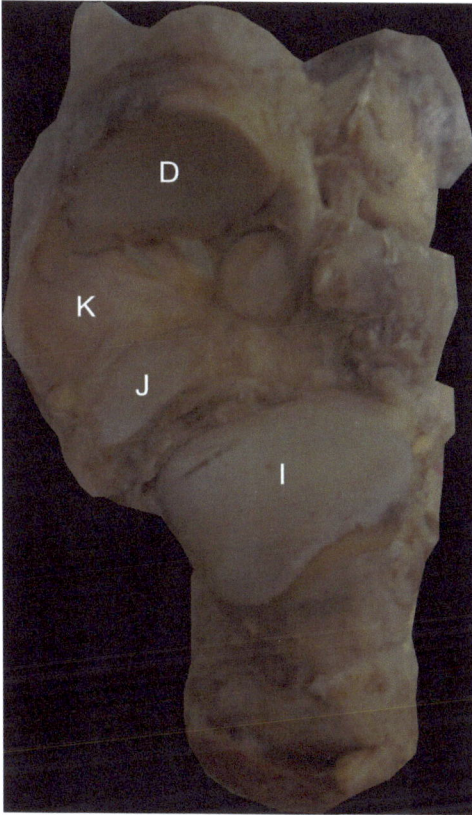

QUESTIONS

1. Name structures I – K.

2. What is structure D?

3. What contributes to the three arches of the foot?

4. What condition commonly afflicts shoe–wearing populations at the lateral aspect of the head of the first metatarsal?

ANSWERS

1. I – subtalar joint; J – sustentaculum tali; K – spring ligament.

2. The plantar aspect of D – navicular.

3. The three arches act as a spring to provide a shock absorbing property and a propulsive mechanism during locomotion. The tarsal bones and their ligamentous attachments form the transverse arch. The peroneus longus tendon also contributes to it. The medial arch is created by the pull of the muscles entering the tarsal tunnel in addition to the tibialis anterior muscle. The lateral aspect of the flexor digitorum longus and brevis muscle contribute to the lateral longitudinal arch. Both the longitudinal arches are also contributed to by the respective sides of the plantar fascia.

4. At this point inappropriate footwear can create an adventitial bursa, which may swell. If there is an associated hallux valgus, arthritis may ensue and form a bunion.

4.16

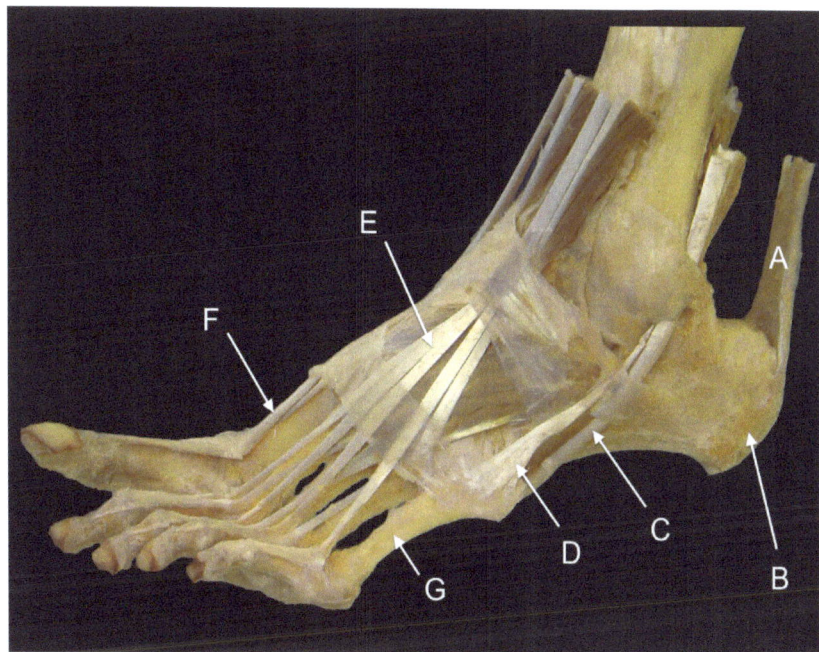

QUESTIONS

1. Identify structures A – G.

2. Describe the bones comprising the tarsometatarsal joint.

3. Which bones comprise the medial and lateral longitudinal arches of the foot?

4. What structures provide support to these longitudinal arches?

5. Describe the Ottawa rules that guide the requirement for X–Rays of the injured foot.

6. What is a Lisfranc fracture–dislocation?

ANSWERS

1. A – Achilles' tendon; B – calcaneus; C – peroneus longus tendon; D – peroneus brevis tendon; E – extensor digitorum longus tendon; F – extensor hallicus longus tendon; G – 5th metatarsal

2. The tarsometatarsal or Lisfranc joint is a plane synovial joint between the three cuneiforms, the cuboid and the bases of the metatarsals.

3. The medial longitudinal arch is comprised of the calcaneus, talus, navicular, cuneiforms and the medial three metarsals.
The lateral longitudinal arch is less pronounced and is comprised of the calcaneus, cuboid and 4th and 5th metatarsals.

4. Ligamentous support to the medial longitudinal arch is provided by spring ligament and ligaments of the articulations between the bones involved. The tendons of tibialis anterior, posterior and peroneus longus, in addition to the plantar aponeurosis, further support the medial arch.

The lateral longitudinal arch is supported by the tendons of fibularis longus and brevis and flexor digitorum muscles, in addition to the long and short plantar ligaments.

5. According to the Ottawa foot rules, an X–Ray of the foot is required if one or more of the following are present:
  – Inability to weight bear both immediately and in the emergency department
  – Bone tenderness at the base of the 5th metatarsal
  – Tenderness over the navicular bone

6. In a Lisfranc fracture dislocation the metatarsals dislocate from their normal articulation with the midtarsal bones. The Lisfranc ligament passes between the medial cuneiform and base of the second metatarsal and is disrupted in this injury.

LOWER LIMB

5 | UPPER LIMB

5.1

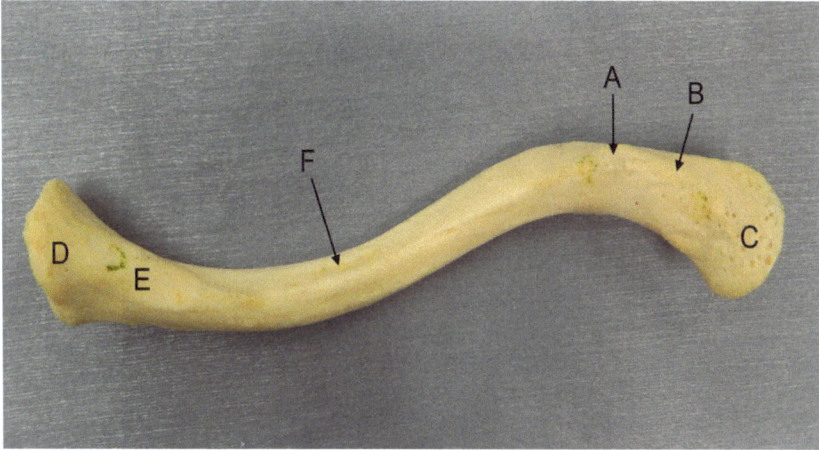

QUESTIONS

1. Identify A – F.

2. Which joint is found at the lateral end of the clavicle? Describe the ligaments that stabilise this joint.

3. The medial head of the clavicle articulates with which bone? What type of joint is present here?

4. Which muscle attaches along line F? What is the function of this muscle?

5. Which nerves pass over the superior border of the clavicle? What are the roots of these nerves?

6. When does ossification of the clavicle begin in fetal life?

7. Which third of the clavicle is most commonly fractured? What structures are at risk in injuries to this area?

ANSWERS

1. A – conoid tubercle; B – trapezoid line; C – acromial end; D – sternal end; E – impression for costoclavicular ligament; F – subclavian groove.

2. The lateral end of the clavicle articulates with the acromion at the acromioclavicular joint. This is a plane synovial joint, which may contain an intra articular disc. The joint is surrounded by a capsule, which is thickened superiorly to form the acromioclavicular ligament.
A strong accessory ligament, the coracoclavicular ligament, passes from the coracoid process of the scapula to the inferior surface of the lateral clavicle. This is separated into two parts named according to their respective shapes; the conoid ligament more medially and trapezoid laterally.

3. The clavicle articulates with the clavicular notch of the manubrium at the sternoclavicular joint. This synovial joint is completely divided by an intra–articular disc.

4. The subclavius muscle originates at the junction of the first rib and its costal cartilage. It passes in a superolateral direction to a groove on the inferior border of the middle third of the clavicle. A minor action of this muscle is depression of the shoulder. In addition it protects the brachial plexus and subclavian vessels following a fracture of the clavicle. Neurovascular injury after clavicular fracture is extremely rare in clinical practice and only occurs in compound injuries, for example a gunshot wound.

5. The supraclavicular nerves pass over the superior border of the clavicle. They can be easily palpated. They arise from cervical nerve roots C3 and C4.

6. Ossification begins during the 5th and 6th weeks of development. It is the first bone to begin ossification in fetal life.

7. 80% of fractures involve the middle third of the clavicle. Structures at risk include the brachial plexus, pleura, and subclavian vessels.

UPPER LIMB

5.2

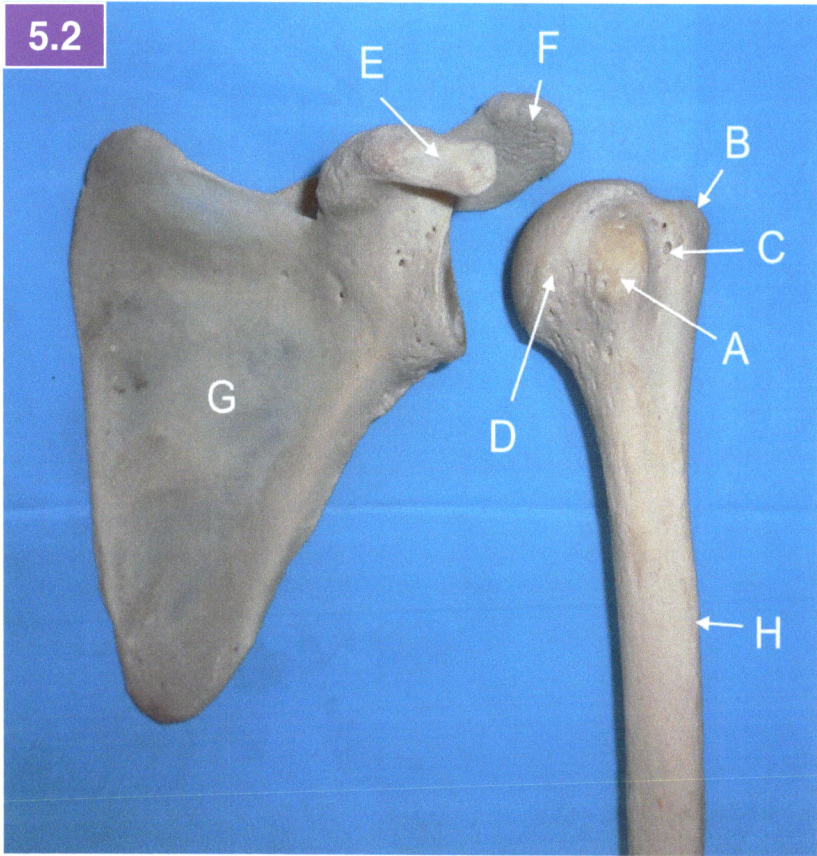

QUESTIONS

1. Identify A – H.

2. Which muscles make up the rotator cuff? Where do they insert on the humerus?

3. What passes through C? Where does this structure originate?

4. What inserts into the infraglenoid tubercle?

5. Where does the deltoid muscle originate and insert? What is its action?

6. What structures contribute to stability at the glenohumeral joint?

7. What is the most common direction of dislocation of the glenohumeral joint?

ANSWERS

1. A – lesser tuberosity; B – greater tuberosity; C – bicipital groove; D – anatomical neck; E – coracoid process; F – acromion; G – subscapular fossa; H – deltoid tuberosity.

2. Supraspinatus, infraspinatus, teres minor and subscapularis. "SITS" is a useful acronym for remembering these. Supraspinatus attaches to the superior portion of the greater tuberosity, infraspinatus to the posterior greater tuberosity, teres minor just below this, and subscapularis attaches to the lesser tuberosity, with its fibers crossing the bicipital groove.

3. The tendon of the long head of biceps brachii. This originates from the supraglenoid tubercle and passes through the joint capsule.

4. The long head of triceps brachii.

5. The origin of the deltoid is the lateral third of the clavicle, the acromion process and the lateral scapular spine. It inserts on the deltoid tuberosity of the humerus. Depending on which part of the deltoid muscle contracts (and therefore the angle of pull), the deltoid can flex, abduct or extend the arm. Broadly speaking, it works in concert with the rotator cuff to elevate the arm away from the trunk.

6. Multiple structures contribute to stability at the glenohumeral joint. These include:
• The glenoid labrum; a fibrocartilagenous tissue that increases the depth of the articulating surface of the glenoid fossa.
• The joint capsule, which extends from the margin of the glenoid fossa to the anatomical neck of the humerus.
• Superior, middle and inferior glenohumeral ligaments.
• Coracohumeral ligament.
• Rotator cuff muscles.
• Biceps Brachii muscle.

7. Anteriorly. Rarely, it may dislocate posteriorly, or inferiorly, the so–called "Luxatio Erecta".

UPPER LIMB

5.3

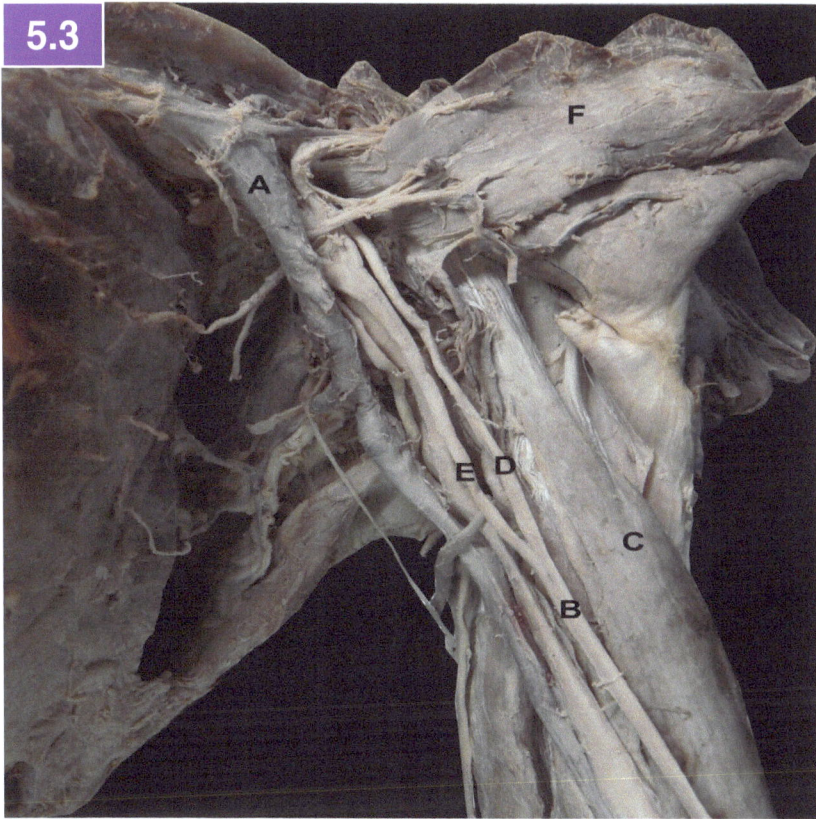

QUESTIONS

1. Identify A – F.

2. Describe the muscles that make up the walls of the axilla.

3. What structures form the boundaries of the axillary inlet?

4. Multiple groups of lymph nodes are found in the axilla. What is their clinical relevance to the surgeon?

5. How can groups of lymph nodes be classified, in relation to surgical dissection of the axilla?

6. During dissection of the axilla, which nerves need to be identified and protected? Which muscles do they supply?

7. What provides the landmark for the termination of the subclavian artery and the origin of the axillary artery?

8. What provides the landmark for the axillary artery becoming the brachial artery?

9. What is the relevance of the pectoralis minor muscle to the axillary artery?

ANSWERS

1. A – axillary vein; B – median nerve; C – biceps brachii muscle; D – lateral cord; E – medial cord; F – pectoralis major muscle (reflected).

2. The axilla is pyramidal in shape with a open base. The anterior wall is made up of pectoralis major, minor and subclavius. The medial wall is formed by the thoracic wall and overlying serratus anterior, the lateral wall consists of the medial border of biceps brachii, coracobrachialis, the humerus and medial border of triceps brachii. Finally, the posterior wall is formed by latissimus dorsi, teres major and minor and subscapularis.

3. The inlet to the axilla is bounded by the first rib, the clavicle, the medial border of the coracoid process and the superior border of the scapula.

4. Axillary lymph nodes are common sites of lymphatic spread from breast cancer.

5. Lymph nodes can be classified into level 1, 2, and 3 according to their position in relation to the pectoralis minor muscle. Level 1 are below, level 2 are behind and level 3 are above the muscle. Typically level 1 and 2 nodes are removed during an axillary dissection.

6. The long thoracic nerve (of Bell) and the thoracodorsal nerve must be protected during axillary surgery. They supply the serratus anterior and latissimus dorsi muscles respectively.

7. The subclavian artery becomes the axillary artery at the lateral margin of the first rib.

8. The axillary artery then becomes the brachial artery at the inferior margin of teres minor.

9. The relationship of the axillary artery to pectoralis minor can, like the lymph nodes, classify it into three parts. The first part is medial to pectoralis minor, the second part is behind pectoralis minor and the third part is lateral to the muscle. At each part the axillary artery gives off 1 (superior thoracic artery), 2 (thoracoacromial artery and lateral thoracic artery) and 3 (anterior and posterior humeral circumflex and the subscapular arteries) branches respectively.

5.4

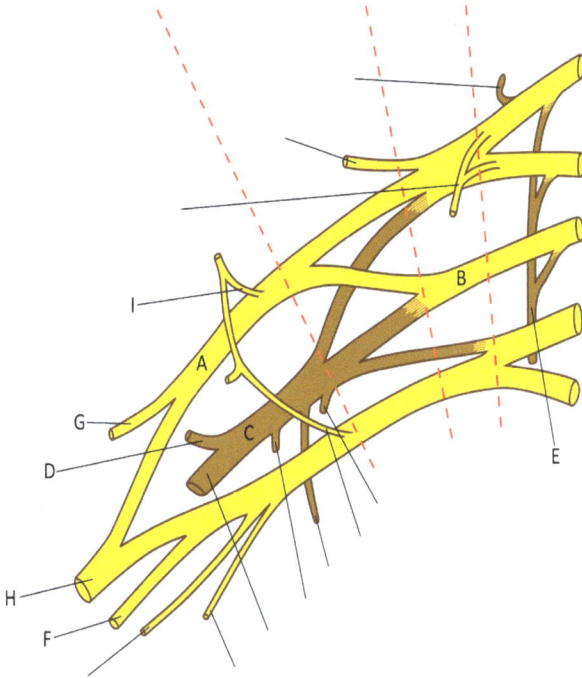

QUESTIONS

1. Identify nerves A – I.

2. Which muscles are supplied by D? What is their action?

3. Which muscles are supplied by G? What is their action?

4. From what nerve roots does the brachial plexus arise?

5. Traction injury to the upper nerve roots of the brachial plexus results in a classic palsy of the upper limb. Name this palsy.

6. What is the most common cause of this palsy?

7. Describe the appearance of the upper limb with this palsy, relating the dysfunction to the nerves and muscles involved.

8. What muscle is supplied by E?

9. What characteristic feature is seen with injury of E?

ANSWERS

1. A – lateral cord; B – middle trunk; C – posterior cord; D – axillary nerve; E – long thoracic nerve; F – ulnar nerve; G – musculocutaneous nerve; H – median nerve; I – lateral pectoral nerve.

2. The axillary nerve supplies the deltoid muscle, which is responsible for elevation of the arm in various planes, depending on which fibers are contracting. The nerve also supplies the teres minor, an external rotator, and the long head of triceps brachii, which extends the elbow.

3. The musculocutaneous nerve supplies the muscles in the anterior compartment of the upper arm: the biceps brachii, brachialis and coracobrachialis. It continues as the lateral cutaneous nerve of the forearm.

4. C5, 6, 7, 8 and T1

5. C5 and C6 nerve root injuries can result in Erb's palsy.

6. This is most commonly caused by shoulder dystocia during difficult labour.

7. This eponymous syndrome produces the so–called waiter's tip position, where the arm is internally rotated at the shoulder, extended at the elbow, with a pronated forearm. This is due to loss of axillary and musculocutaneous nerve function, paralysing the external rotators of the shoulder and flexors and supinators of the forearm.

8. E is the long thoracic nerve, which supplies serratus anterior.

9. Serratus anterior attaches the deep aspect of the scapula to the thoracic wall. Paralysis causes winging of the scapula, most evident when the patient is asked to push against a wall.

UPPER LIMB

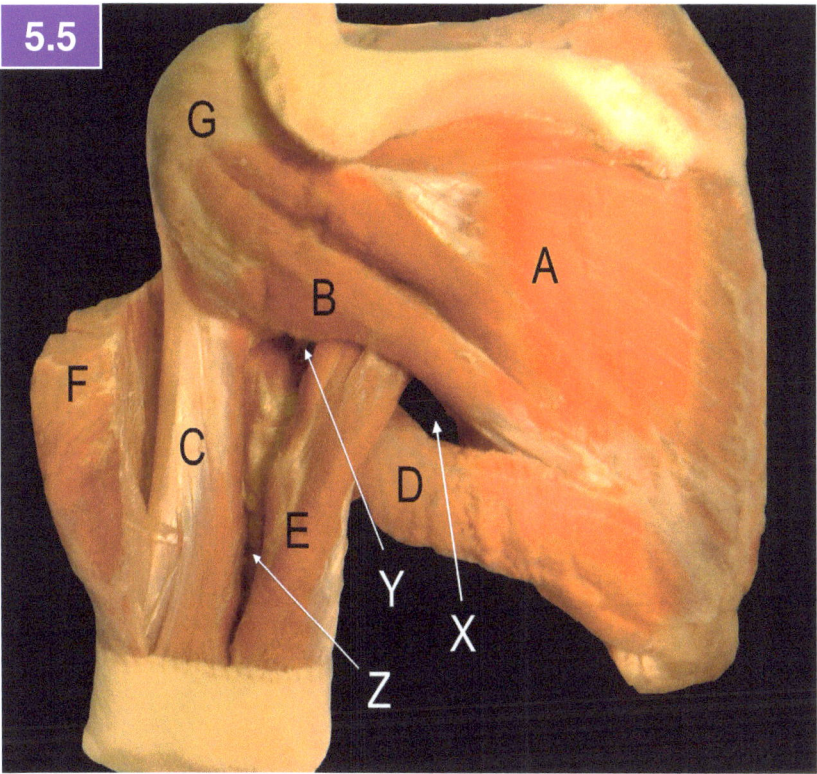

QUESTIONS

1. Name the structures labelled A – G on this posterior view of the shoulder.

2. Which of these contribute to the rotator cuff? Which other muscles not seen here are part of the rotator cuff?

3. What are the openings shown by X, Y and Z?

4. Name one structure that passes through each one.

5. With which bony structure does G articulate? What joint does this form, and what articulations are possible here?

6. Which muscle, passing below D, forms the remainder of the posterior wall of the axilla? What is its innervation?

ANSWERS

1. A – infraspinatus; B – teres minor; C – lateral head of triceps; D – teres major; E – long head of triceps; F – deltoid (cut); G – head of humerus.

2. The infraspinatus and teres minor for the posterior part of the rotator cuff, along with the supraspinatus (superior) and subscapularis (anterior)

3. X is the triangular space or medial triangular space; Y is the quadrangular space and Z is the triangular interval.

4. The scapular circumflex vessels pass through the triangular space, the axillary nerve and posterior humeral circumflex artery pass though the quadrangular space and the radial nerve and profunda brachii artery pass through the lateral triangular interval.

5. The humeral head articulates with the glenoid fossa of the scapula, forming the glenohumeral joint. Flexion, extension, abduction, adduction, internal and external rotation and circumduction are possible at this joint.

6. The latissimus dorsi passes below teres major to attach to the floor of the intertubercular groove of the humerus. It is innervated by the thoracodorsal nerve.

5.6

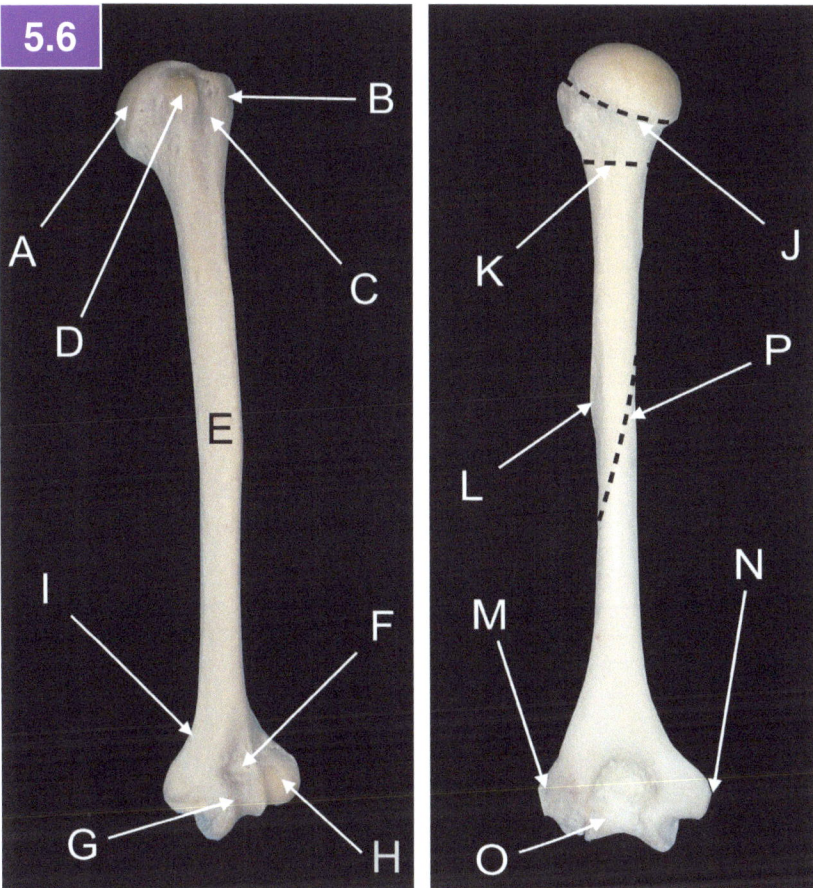

QUESTIONS

1. Label A – P.

2. What structure is at risk in a fractured surgical neck of humerus and which population demographic is likely to suffer from this fracture?

3. How does one test the function of this nerve?

4. What structure will be at risk from a mid–shaft fracture?

5. What lies posterior to the medial epicondyle?

6. How will you assess the function of this structure?

7. If damage to this nerve occurs at the wrist, what will be observed?

ANSWERS

1. A – humeral head; B – greater tuberosity; C – intertubercular groove; D – lesser tuberosity; E – shaft; F – coronoid fossa; G – trochlea; H – capitellum; I – medial supracondylar ridge; J – anatomical neck; K – surgical neck; L – deltoid tuberosity; M – lateral epicondyle; N – medial epicondyle; O – olecranon fossa; P – spiral groove.

2. The surgical neck has a reduced density of mineralised bone post–menopause. For this reason, fractures of this area usually occur in elderly osteoporotic females. The axillary nerve arises from the posterior trunk of the brachial plexus and leaves the quadrangular space to enter the deltoid muscle. This comes in very close contact to the surgical neck and a fracture may damage the nerve

3. The axillary nerve has dual sensory and motor function. It provides sensation to the so called "regimental badge area", on the superolateral portion of the arm over the inferior portion of the deltoid muscle. It provides motor fibres to the deltoid and teres minor muscles.

4. Fractures at the mid–shaft usually involve the spiral groove, which is formed as the radial nerve grooves around the posterior aspect of the arm. Therefore a fracture at this site may result in radial nerve palsy.

5. The ulnar nerve is a branch of the medial cord of the brachial plexus and descends down the medial aspect of the forearm and passes under the medial epicondyle to pierce the flexor carpi ulnaris muscle.

6. The nerve supplies the flexor carpi ulnaris muscle, medial half of the flexor digitorum profundus muscle and all the intrinsic muscles of the hand except for the lateral two lumbricals and the thenar muscles. Its sensory supply is to the little finger and half of the ring finger. To assess its motor function one may assess strength of the adducted fingers by placing a paper in between the fingers and asking the patient to resist it being pulled away from them.

7. A nerve injury at this point will result in clawing of the fourth and fifth digit. This occurs due to loss of action of the medial two lumbricals. This muscle flexes the digits at the MCP joint whilst extending at the PIP and DIP joint. As there is a loss of action of this muscle the extensor digitorum holds the digits extended at the MCP joint but the unaffected long flexors of the forearm flex the digits at the PIP and DIP joints. Clawing of the digits does not occur in a proximal lesion as the long flexors are also paralysed, leaving the digits in extension.

5.7

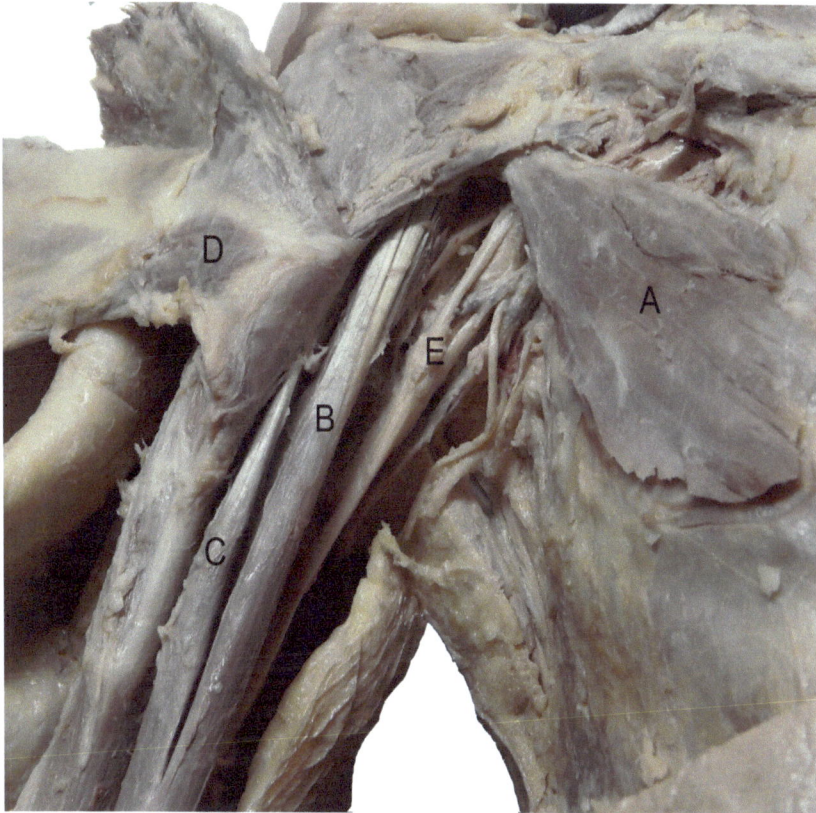

QUESTIONS

1. Name structures A – E.

2. Describe the compartments of the arm.

3. Which structures form the apex of the axilla? What passes through this canal?

4. What is the insertion point of muscle B? What movement occurs following contraction of this muscle?

5. What clinical feature is found following rupture of the long head of biceps brachii?

6. Which nerve supplies sensation to the medial border of the upper arm? How may this nerve be damaged?

ANSWERS

1. A – pectoralis minor; B – short head of biceps brachii; C – long head of biceps brachii; D – pectoralis major (reflected) E – median nerve.

2. The arm is separated into two muscular compartments by the lateral and medial intermuscular septum. The anterior compartment contains the flexor muscles; biceps brachii, coracobrachialis and brachialis. The posterior compartment contains the triceps brachii and anconeus muscles.

3. The following structures form the superior border of the axilla: the lateral border of the first rib, the medial border of the coracoid process, the superior border of the scapula and the posterior border of the clavicle.

The axillary artery, vein and nerve of the brachial plexus pass through the canal formed by these structures.

4. The tendon of biceps brachii inserts onto the radial tuberosity. The bicipital aponeurosis inserts into the deep fascia of the forearm and offers some protection to the structures in the antecubital fossa. The biceps is a powerful supinator of the forearm. It also flexes the elbow joint and assists in shoulder flexion.

5. Rupture of biceps tendon leads to bunching of the muscle within the arm, also known as Popeye's sign. Ruptures of the proximal or distal tendons may occur, but a distal rupture produces far more disability and necessitates surgical repair.

6. The intercostobrachial nerve from T2, supplies the medial border of the upper arm. It is an extension of the second intercostal nerve. It may be injured during axillary node clearance following breast cancer.

UPPER LIMB

5.8

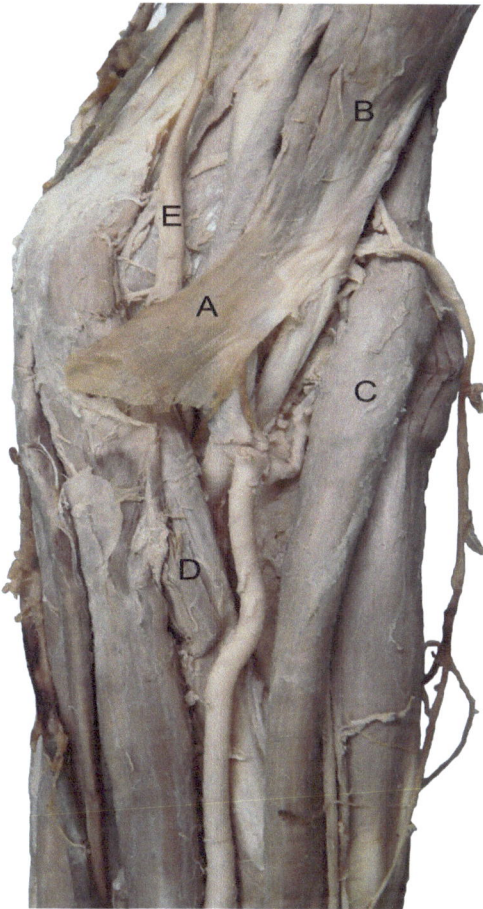

QUESTIONS

1. Name structures A – E. Where does structure A insert?

2. Describe the borders of the antecubital fossa.

3. From medial to lateral, describe its contents.

4. What structures form the roof of the antecubital fossa?

5. Bifurcation of which nerve may also be found at its lateral border? Name the branches.

6. Which nerve passes posterior to the medial epicondyle? Describe the path of this nerve through the forearm.

7. What is Volkmann's ischaemic contracture?

ANSWERS

1. A – bicipital aponeurosis; B – biceps brachii; C – brachioradialis; D – pronator teres; E – median nerve.

The biceps tendon inserts on radial tuberosity. The bicipital aponeurosis passes across biceps brachii and the median nerve and fuses with the deep fascia covering the origin of the flexor muscles of the forearm

2. The borders of the antecubital fosssa are as follows:

Lateral: medial border of brachioradialis
Medial: lateral border of pronator teres
Superior: horizontal line drawn between the medial and lateral epicondyles of the humerus

3. Median nerve, brachial artery, tendon of biceps brachii.

4. Skin and superficial fascia including the antecubital vein.

5. Radial nerve, superficial and deep branches.

6. Ulnar nerve. This passes down the medial border of the forearm between flexor carpi ulnaris and flexor digitorum profundus.

7. This is permanent fibrous contraction of the forearm flexor muscles that occurs as a consequence of inadequate perfusion from the brachial artery. Most commonly caused by a supracondylar fracture of the humerus.

UPPER LIMB

5.9

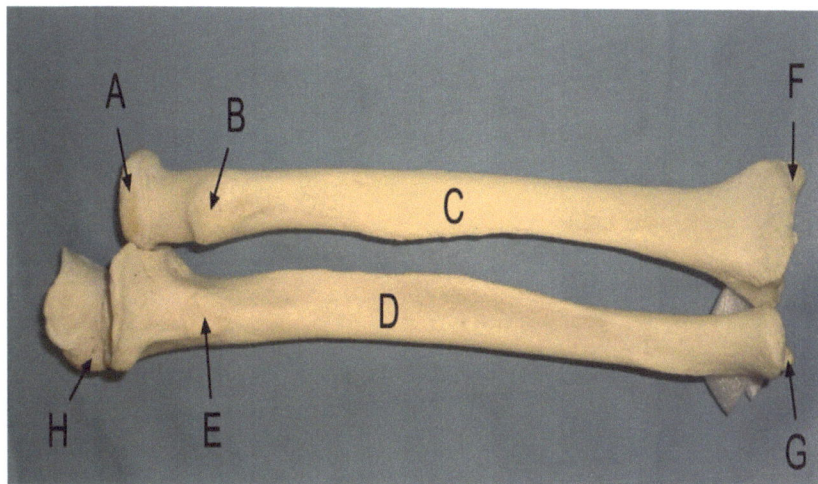

QUESTIONS

1. Label structures A – H.

2. The tendon of which muscle inserts on the radial tuberosity? What structure blends with the deep fascia covering the anterior compartment of the forearm?

3. What ligament maintains the stability of the proximal radio–ulnar joint? How is this articulation related to the elbow joint?

4. Which muscle originates at the medial epicondyle of the humerus and along the oblique line of the radius? Describe the insertion of this muscle.

5. What pattern of injury is found in a Galeazzi fracture? How does this differ from a Monteggia fracture?

6. What eponymous name is give to a fracture of the distal radius with dorsal and radial displacement of the wrist and hand?

UPPER LIMB

ANSWERS

1. A – radial head; B – radial tuberosity;   C – radial shaft; D – ulna shaft; E – tuberosity of ulna F – radial styloid; G – ulnar styloid; H – olecranon of ulna.

2. The tendon of biceps brachii. The bicipital aponeurosis diverges from the biceps tendon and blends with the deep fascia on the anterior forearm. It provides some protection to the underlying brachial artery and median nerve.

3. The annular ligament attaches to the anterior and posterior margins of the radial notch. It allows free rotation of the radius. The capsule of the elbow joint is consistent with that of the proximal radio–ulnar joint.

4. Flexor digitorum superficialis. The tendons pass below the flexor retinaculum, through the carpal tunnel to insert on the middle phalanges of the index, middle, ring and little fingers.

5. Galeazzi fracture, fracture of the radius with dislocation of the distal radioulnar joint. A Monteggia fracture, fracture of the proximal ulna with dislocation of the head of the radius.

6. Colles' fracture. A "dinner fork" deformity is often noted. Originally described by Abraham Colles on clinical findings alone.

5.10

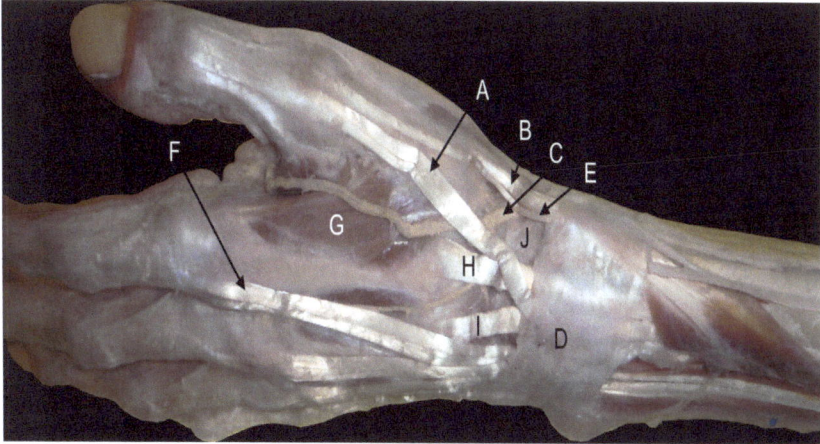

QUESTIONS

1. Name structures A – I and the anatomical area marked J.

2. Describe the extensor compartments of the wrist.

3. What are the borders of the anatomical snuffbox?

4. How would you test for a fracture of the scaphoid?

5. Name one complication of a fracture of the scaphoid.

6. Where do the extensors of the forearm receive their innervation? Which muscle does this pierce?

7. Pain over the anterior tendons of the snuffbox with flexion of the thumb while the wrist is in ulnar deviation is suggestive of which condition?

ANSWERS

1. A – extensor pollicis longus; B – extensor pollicis brevis; C – radial artery; D – extensor retinaculum; E – abductor pollicis longus; F – extensor digitorum; G – first dorsal interosseous; H – extensor carpi radialis longus; I – extensor carpi radialis brevis; J – anatomical snuff box.

2. There are six extensor compartments of the wrist. Compartment one contains the abductor pollicis longus and extensor pollicis brevis muscle. Compartment two contains the extensor carpi radialis longus and brevis. The third compartment contains extensor pollicis longus. Compartment four contains the tendons of extensor indicis and extensor digitorum. Compartment five transmits the tendon of extensor digiti minimi. The final compartment is for the extensor carpi ulnaris muscle.

3. The anterior compartment is formed from the tendons of extensor pollicis brevis and abductor pollicis longus. The posterior boundary is formed from the extensor pollicis longus tendons.

4. To test for a fracture of the scaphoid, one must palpate the bone within the anatomical snuffbox and also load the bone by compressing the thumb into the carpus. The scaphoid tubercle can be palpated on the anterior aspect of the wrist, 1 cm distal to the wrist crease on the radial side. Pain across the scaphoid bone would suggest a fracture.

5. A fracture may result in avascular necrosis. The scaphoid bone receives its blood supply distally and fractures of this bone may result in avascular necrosis. Patients will require a follow–up X–ray two weeks post injury to allow for any fracture to reveal itself.

6. The radial nerve innervates the brachioradialis muscle and all the rest are innervated by the posterior interosseous nerve (a branch of the deep radial nerve). The posterior interosseous nerve emerges from the supinator muscle roughly one hands–breadth below the elbow joint.

7. Pain over the anterior boundary of the snuffbox, whilst in this position suggests an inflammation of the tendon. This condition is called De Quervain's tenosynovitis, caused through repetitive strain. The test is called Finkelstein's test.

5.11

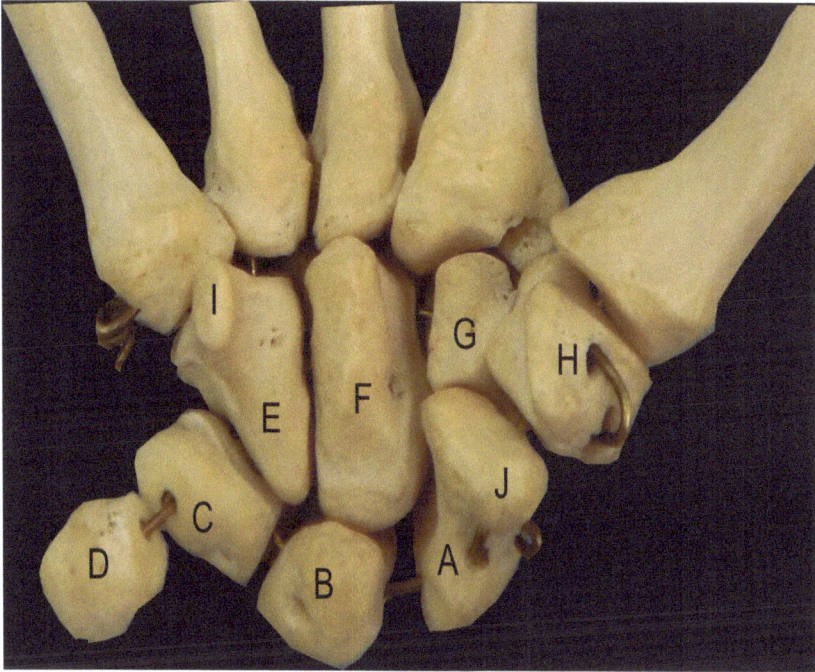

QUESTIONS

1. Name the structures labelled A – J.

2. Which carpal bone may dislocate with a fall onto the outstretched hand?

3. What type of bone is the pisiform and within what structure does it run?

4. The ulnar nerve runs through Guyon's canal, what forms the roof of this structure?

5. The flexor retinaculum form the roof of which tunnel? What are its attachments?

6. Which structures pass through this tunnel?

7. What symptoms are classically described by the patient suffering with carpal tunnel syndrome?

ANSWERS

1. A – scaphoid; B – lunate; C – triquetrum; D – pisiform; E – hamate; F – capitate; G – trapezoid; H – trapezium; I – hook of the hamate; J – scaphoid tubercle.

2. The lunate bone sits in the proximal row of carpal bones and acts as a cup for the large capitate to sit in. A fall on the outstretched hand may result in a peri–lunate dislocation, which would be confirmed by a lateral X–ray view of the wrist.

3. The pisiform bone is part of the proximal row of carpal bones and is found in the tendon of flexor carpi ulnaris. It can therefore be described as a sesamoid bone.

4. Guyon's canal transmits the ulnar nerve and ulnar artery. The roof is made up of the palmer carpal ligament and the floor by the flexor retinaculum. Compression of this nerve occurs whilst gripping the handlebar of a bike.

5. The flexor retinaculum attaches from the pisiform and hamate and travels to insert into the tubercle of the scaphoid and trapezium.

6. The tunnel transmits nine tendons and one nerve. The nerve is the median nerve and the tendons include the four tendons of flexor digitorum superficialis, the four tendons of flexor carpi profundus and the tendon of flexor pollicis longus. A small slip of ligament is given off to separate the flexor carpi radialis tendon from the carpal tunnel.

7. Paraesthesia in the first, second, third and lateral half of the fourth digits of the hand, typically at night. These symptoms can be elicited using Tinel's test and Phalen's test. Both of these tests act to worsen the compression of the nerve and therefore elicit the patient's symptoms.

UPPER LIMB

5.12

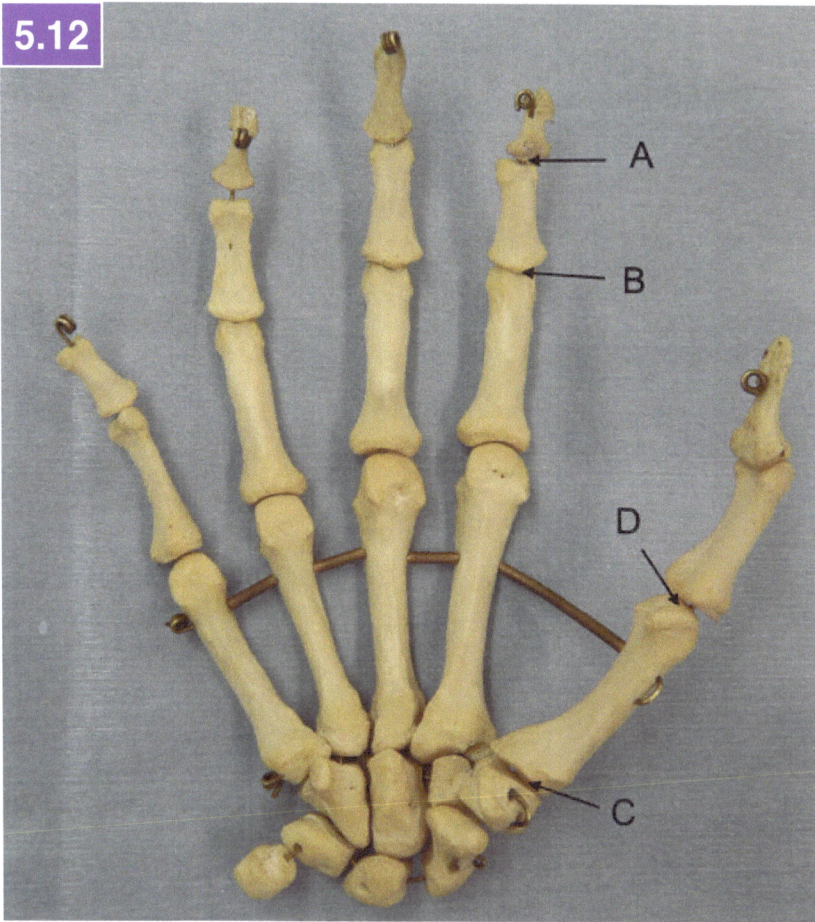

QUESTIONS

1. Name the joints labelled A – D.

2. What type of joint is C? What movements are permitted at this joint?

3. Describe a Bennett's fracture. What is the common mechanism of injury?

4. What is the eponymous name given to the bony swellings that can develop in the distal interphalangeal joints? What clinical condition are they associated with?

5. Which bone(s) are most commonly involved in a boxer's fracture?

6. What are Bouchard's nodes and where are they found?

ANSWERS

1. A – distal interphalangeal joint; B – proximal interphalangeal joint; C – first carpometacarpal joint, also know as trapeziometacarpal joint; D – metacarpophalangeal joint.

2. The first carpometacarpal joint is a saddle-type synovial joint that permits flexion, extension, abduction, adduction and circumduction.

3. Fracture of the base of the first metacarpal that extends into the 1st CMC joint. Most commonly caused by axial loading of the 1st metacarpal while in partial flexion e.g. when punching a firm object or falling onto the thumb.

4. Heberden's nodes. Named after William Heberden. A sign of osteoarthritis.

5. Fracture through the neck of the 5th metacarpal is the classic boxer's fracture, cause by axial loading of that bone typically when a punch is landed against an unforgiving object.

6. Bony outgrowths or cysts found on the proximal interphalageal joints, associated with rheumatoid arthritis.

5.13

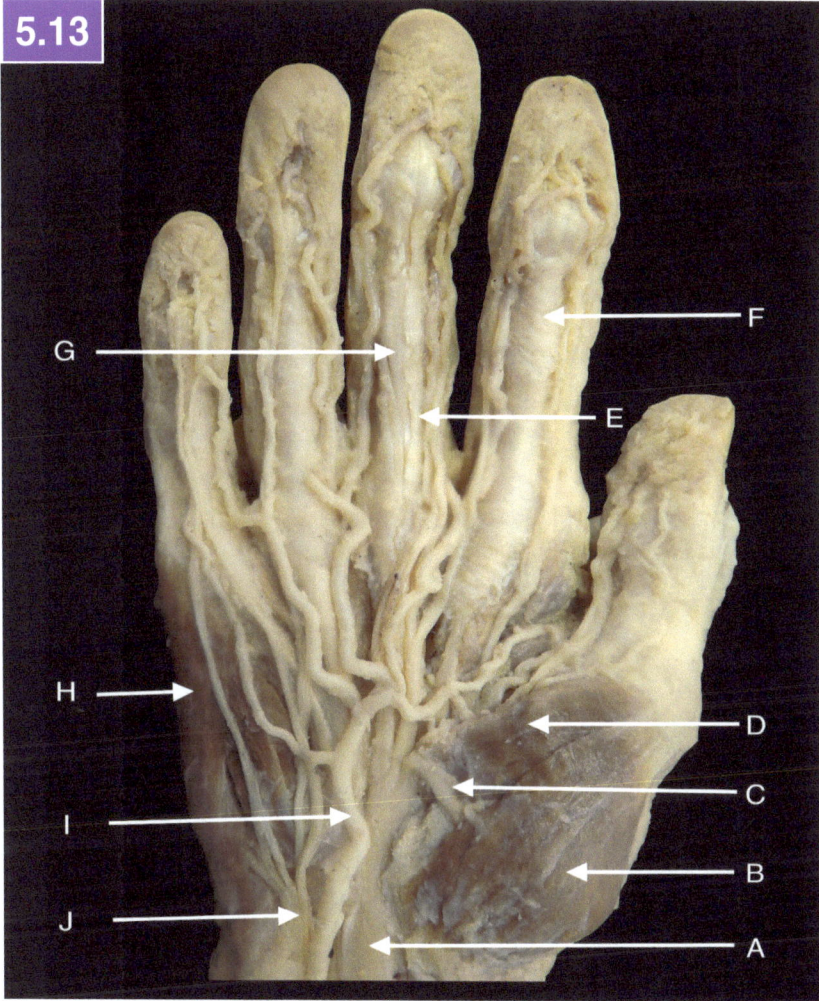

QUESTIONS

1. Name structures A – J.
2. Describe the innervation of the muscles of the hand.
3. What are the hypothenar muscles?
4. What are the functions of the interossei muscles?
5. What action do the lumbricals perform?
6. Describe the dorsal expansion.
7. Describe the clinical relevance of the flexor tendon sheath.

UPPER LIMB

ANSWERS

1. A – median nerve; B – abductor pollicis brevis; C – recurrent branch of the median nerve; D – opponens pollicis; E – tendon of flexor digitorum superficialis; F – Flexor tendon sheath; G – tendon of flexor digitorum profundus; H – abductor digiti minimi; I – ulnar artery; J – ulnar nerve.

2. The musculature of the hand primarily receives its innervation from the median and ulnar nerve. The median nerve is said to innervate the "LOAF" muscles, which are the radial two lumbricals, opponens pollices, abductor pollices brevis and flexor pollicis brevis. The ulnar nerve innervates the hypothenar muscles, interossei, the medial two lumbricals and adductor pollicis.

3. The hypothenar muscles all serve the little finger and are complementary to the thenar muscles. They are flexor digiti minimi, opponens digiti minimi, and abductor digiti minimi.

4. The interossei can be divided into two parts; palmer and dorsal. The dorsal part abducts the finger and palmer parts adduct the fingers. The middle finger abducts and cannot adduct. This is because the midline of the hand runs down the middle finger, therefore it only possess a dorsal interossei.

5. The lumbricals are intrinsic muscles of the hand that arise from the flexor digitorum tendons and the palmar aspect of the hand. They insert into the dorsal expansion. Contraction of this muscle will extend the proximal interphalangeal (PIP) and distal interphalangeal (DIP) joints, while flexing the finger at the MCPJ. They act on fingers two to five.

6. As the extensor digitorum tendons approach the MCPJ, a connective tissue starts to form around the joint and tendon, this is the beginning of the extensor hood. This then splits, allowing for two bands to form on either side of the digit, which insert into both the lateral edges of the middle phalanx and the base of the dorsal aspect of the DIPJ.

7. The flexor tendon sheath is a fibrous sheath with contains a synovial lining that lubricates the flexor tendons as they are transmitted to the appropriate phalanx. This space is important as a cellulitis of the finger can spread to the flexor sheath and since the sheath is continuous with the fascia of the palm and forearm allow the infection to ascend up the arm.
The flexor tendon sheath should be considered a closed fascial compartment, where a compartment syndrome may develop as inflammation worsens. As a result, infections within the sheath should be treated with emergency incision and irrigation.

5.14

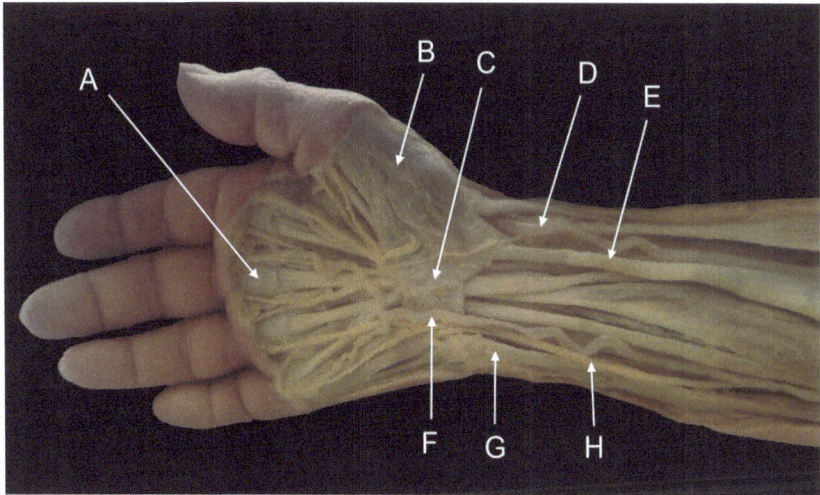

QUESTIONS

1. Label A – H.
2. What are the borders of the carpal tunnel?
3. What structures pass through the carpal tunnel?
4. Which nerve passes superficial to the flexor retinaculum?
5. What are the common symptoms of carpal tunnel syndrome?
6. What conditions is it associated with?
7. Describe how you might investigate and manage this condition.

UPPER LIMB

ANSWERS

1. A – A1 pulley; B – abductor pollicis in thenar eminence; C – transverse palmar ligament; D – radial artery; E – flexor carpi radialis; F – ulnar artery; G – flexor carpi ulnaris; H – ulnar nerve.

2. The borders of the carpal tunnel are as follows:

Superficial:	Flexor retinaculum
Deep:	Proximal row of carpal bones
Medial:	Hook of hamate and pisiform
Lateral:	Scaphoid tubercle and trapezium

3. The contents of the carpal tunnel include the four tendons of flexor digitorum profundus, the four tendons of flexor digitorum superficialis, the tendon of flexor pollicis longus and the median nerve. The tendon of flexor carpi radialis is surrounded by the lateral portion of the flexor retinaculum.

4. The palmar cutaneous branch of the median nerve begins proximal to the flexor retinaculum. As it passes superficial to the retinaculum it divides into lateral and medial branches.

5. Symptoms of carpal tunnel syndrome include pain, numbness, tingling, weakness and clumsiness in the sensory distribution of the median nerve, which includes the lateral three digits and lateral half of the fourth digit. Symptoms are often worse at night and are provoked by activities that involve flexion and extension of the wrist, or raising the arms.

6. The syndrome is often associated with other conditions, including the following: hypothyroidism, rheumatoid arthritis, pregnancy and acromegaly.

7. Tinel's test involves tapping over the carpal tunnel. Phalen's test involves the examiner holding the patient's wrist in full flexion for one minute. Both tests are positive if they reproduce the patient's symptoms. Neither are particularly sensitive nor specific. Typically patients with suspected carpal tunnel syndrome will undergo nerve conduction testing to demonstrate the site of the compression, as the medial nerve can be compressed at other points along its course, including by the pronator teres muscle. Management may be conservative, including activity modification and night splinting; medical, including steroid injections; and surgical, typically a carpal tunnel decompression by dividing the carpal ligament.

UPPER LIMB

6 SPINE

SPINE

6.1

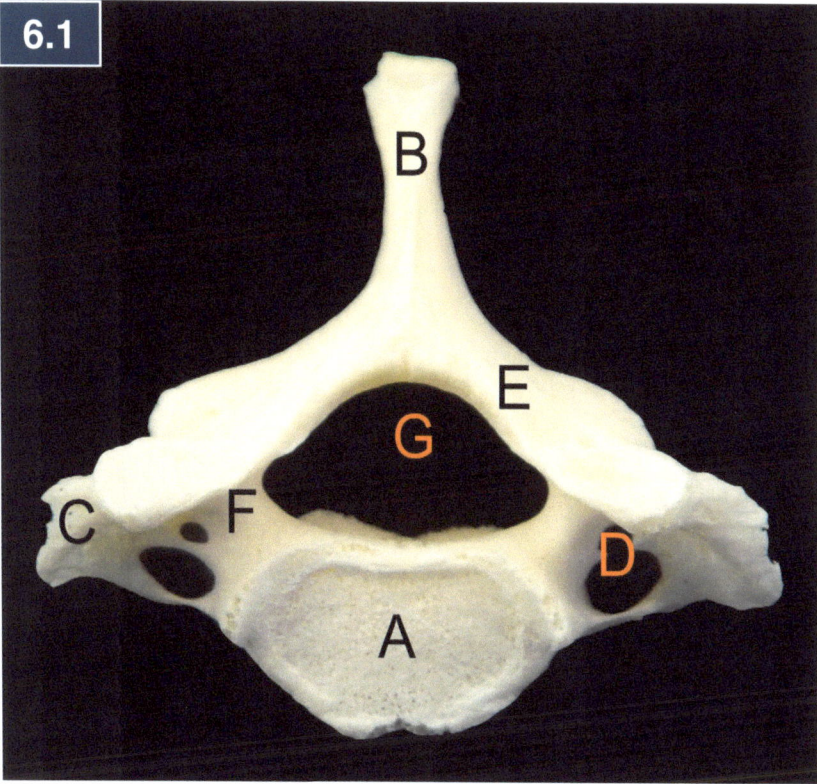

QUESTIONS

1. Name structures A – G.
2. Which structure passes through D?
3. Which vertebrae is this most likely to be?
4. What is found within G?
5. The vertebral arch is formed by which structures?
6. Describe the joints found between vertebrae.
7. What ligamentous structures pass between the vertebral bodies?
8. What is found between the bodies of vertebrae? What layers are they separated into and of what are they comprised?

SPINE

ANSWERS

1. A – vertebral body; B – spinous process; C – transverse process; D – foramen transversarium; E – lamina; F – pedicle; G – vertebral foramen.

2. Vertebral artery. These are branches of the subclavian artery and enter the foramen transversarium at the level of the 6th cervical vertebrae.

3. C7 the vertebra prominens. Demonstrated by its prominent spinous process. Unlike other cervical vertebrae this is not bifid.

4. Spinal cord, meninges, anterior and posterior spinal arteries, spinal veins, internal vertebral venous plexus.

5. Vertebral laminae and pedicles.

6. Six joints in total. Two superior facet joints. Two inferior facet joints. Two secondary cartilaginous joints between the vertebral body and vertebral disc above and below.

7. The anterior and posterior longitudinal ligaments. The anterior longitudinal ligament passes from the base of the occiput to the front of the upper sacrum. The posterior longitudinal ligament extends from the body of C2 to the sacrum, it is continuous with the tectorial membrane above.

8. Intervertebral discs are found connecting the vertebrae. They consist of an outer annulus fibrosus of fibrocartilage and an inner nucleus pulposus comprised of collagen fibers in a mucoprotein gel, rich in polysaccharides.

SPINE

6.2

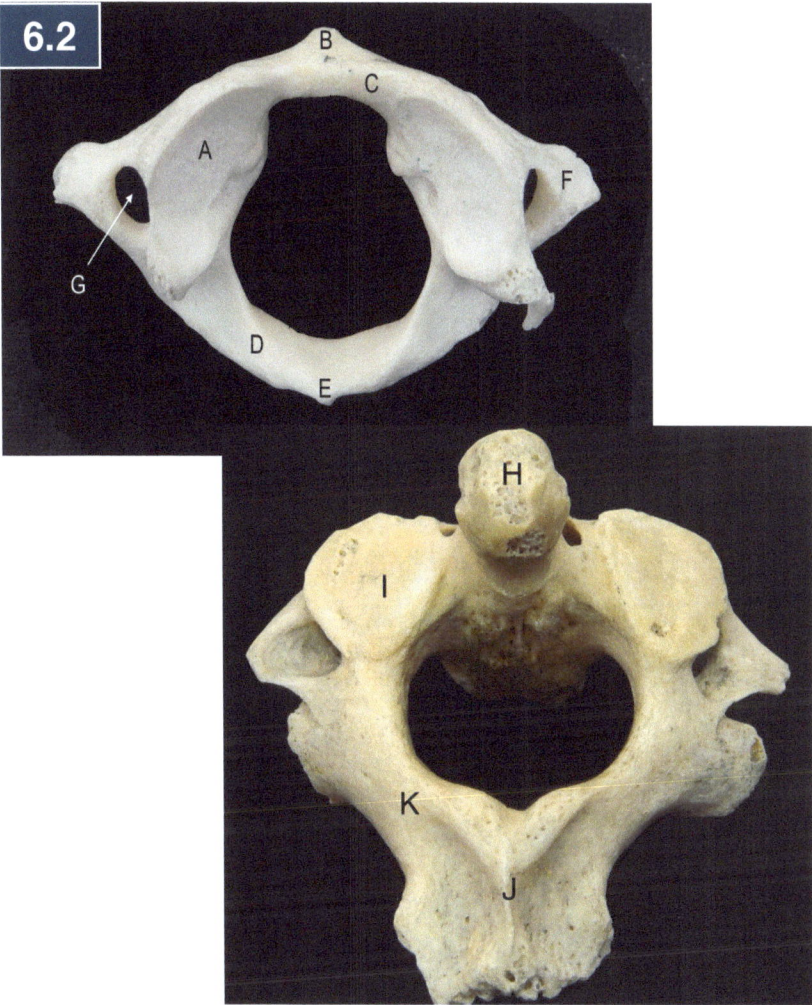

QUESTIONS

1. Which vertebrae are these?
2. Name structures A – K.
3. Why are these considered atypical vertebrae?
4. What structures comprise the atlantoaxial joint?
5. What movements are permitted between these vertebrae and the skull?
6. What mechanism may lead to a fracture of H?
7. What factors might predispose to subluxation between these two vertebrae?

SPINE

ANSWERS

1. The first and second cervical vertebrae, also known as the atlas and axis, are shown in the image. The first cervical vertebrae is names "atlas" after the Greek Titan, who supported the sky as C1 supports the skull.

2. A – superior articulating facet; B – anterior tubercle; C – anterior arch; D – posterior arch; E – posterior tubercle; F – transverse process; G – foramen transversarium; H – dens; I – superior articulating facet; J – spinous process (bifid); K – lamina.

3. The structure of these vertebrae is unusual in comparison to the other cervical vertebrae. The atlas is a ring, comprised of anterior and posterior arches, which are separated by the lateral bodies. These bony expansions provide the surfaces for articulation with the skull. It has no vertebral body; this has been "stolen" by the axis to form the bony protrusion known as the dens.

The axis sits below the atlas, its large, round, superior articular surfaces articulate with the atlas. It has thick, strong laminae and short transverse processes. The dens protrudes up through the ring of the atlas.

4. The atlantoaxial joint is comprised of median and lateral articulations.
The median articulation is between the dens and the posterior surface of the anterior arch of the atlas. This is a synovial pivot joint and is supported posteriorly by the transverse ligament of the atlas, which passes between the lateral masses of the atlas.
The lateral articulations are gliding synovial joints between the lateral bodies of the atlas above and the superior facets of the axis below.

5. The primary movement at the atlanto–occipital joint is flexion, in addition to a degree of lateral flexion and rotation.

6. Loading in flexion is the mot common cause of a fractured dens. They are classified by Anderson & D'Alonzo (1974) into three types, with progressively decreasing levels of stability.

7. Atlanto–axial subluxation should be considered not only in a trauma setting, but also as a source of airway compromise in patients receiving a general anaesthetic. Predisposing conditions include; rheumatoid arthritis, ankylosing spondylitis, Down's syndrome and Marfan's disease.

SPINE

6.3

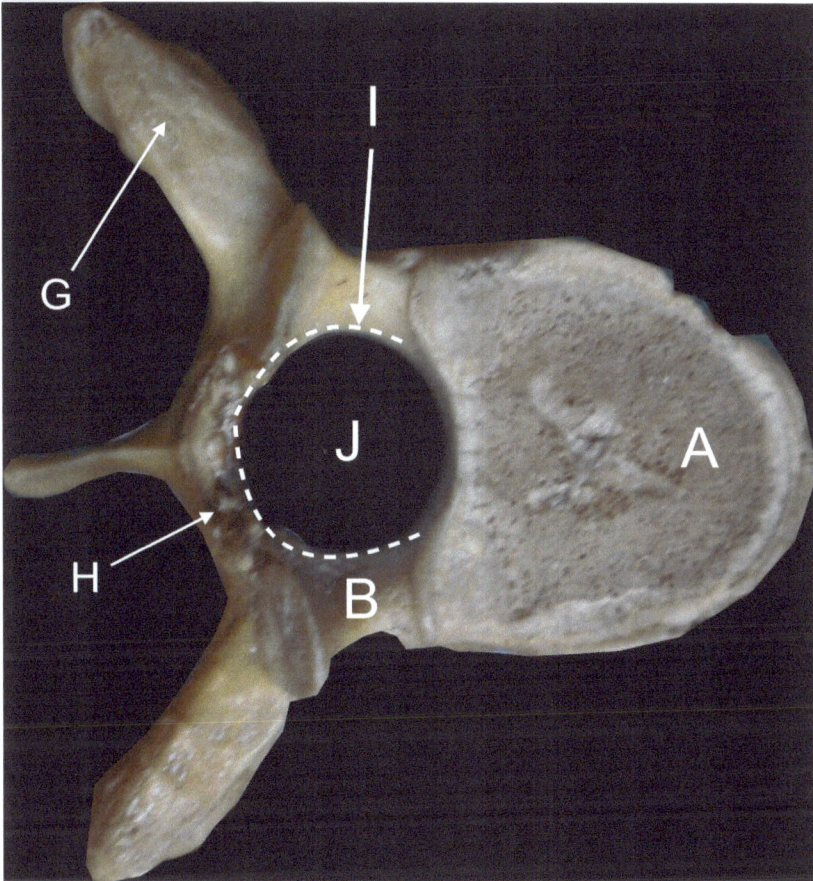

QUESTIONS

1. Label A and B.
2. How do the spinal nerves leave the spinal column?
3. Describe how the ribs articulate with the vertebrae.
4. Which way does the articulating disc herniate? Why is this?
5. Label G – J.

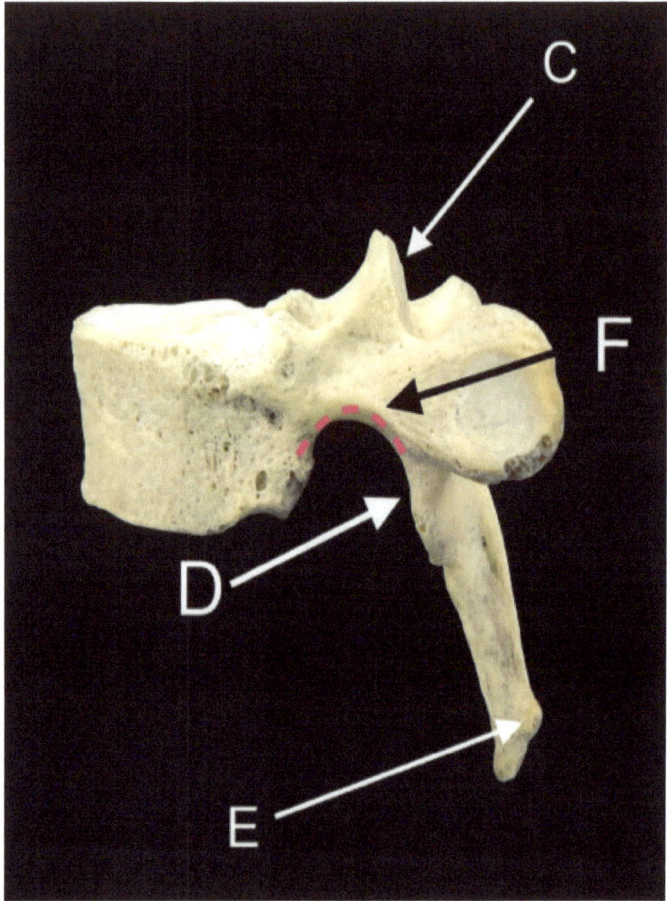

QUESTIONS

6. Label C – F.

7. Describe the appearance of the spinous processes of thoracic verte-brae.

8. At which thoracic level is the carina found? What other structures are found at this level?

ANSWERS

1. A – vertebral body; B – pedicle.

2. In the thoracic region the spinal nerve is formed from incoming sensory fibers and outgoing motor fibers. This spinal nerve exits via the inferior aspect of its respective vertebra through the intervertebral foramen. For example, T5 leaves underneath the fifth thoracic pedicle.

3. The head of each rib has two articulating facets. One facet articulates with the body of the vertebra above and the other with the body of the vertebra below. The neck also has an area that articulates with the transverse process of its respective vertebra.

4. The intervertebral discs are secondary cartilaginous joints of the fibrocartilaginous variety. Anteriorly they are bound by the anterior longitudinal ligament and posterior longitudinal ligament on the anterior and posterior wall respectively of the vertebral body, within the spinal canal. The area of least support is in the posterolateral position, where the intervertebral disc herniates, therefore putting the spinal nerves at risk of being compressed.

5. G – transverse process; H – lamina; I – vertebral arch; J – spinal canal.

6. C – superior articular facet; D – inferior articular facet; E – spinous process; F – intervertebral foramen.

7. The spinous processes of thoraic vertebrae are long and inferior sloping. The lower thoracic vertebrae have shorter, broader spinous processes as they become progressively more lumbarised.

8. The carina is found at the level of T4. This is a very important level as it corresponds to key anatomical events. These include the start and finish of the arch of the aorta, the azygos vein draining into the SVC, the origin of the recurrent laryngeal nerve and the level of the sternal angle which separates the superior and inferior mediastinum.

SPINE

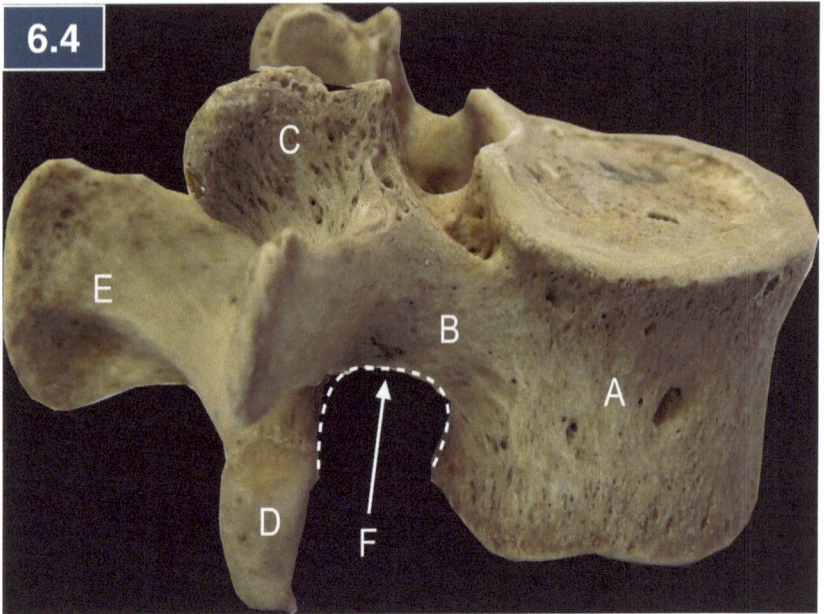

QUESTIONS

1. Label A – F.

2. Describe a typical lumbar vertebra.

3. How do the facet joints articulate at the lumbar region? How does this relate to the movements permitted in this region?

4. What is spondylolisthesis?

5. How does L1 differ from L5?

6. What will occur if a vertebral body shows asymmetry?

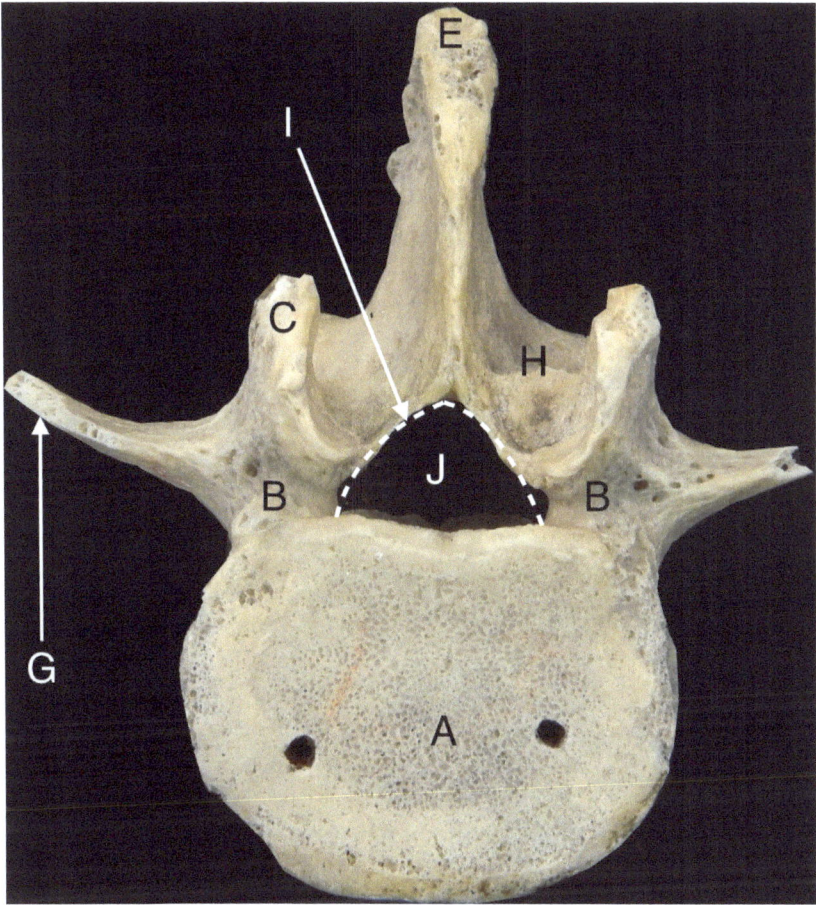

QUESTIONS

7. Label G – J.

8. What type of joint is found along the spine?

9. What level does the spinal cord end in adults and children?

10. What are the symptoms of cauda equina syndrome?

11. What herniates in a disc herniation?

12. Describe the ligamentous support of the lumbar vertebra.

13. Which structures lie in the extradural space?

SPINE

ANSWERS

1. A – vertebral body; B – pedicle; C – superior articulating facet; D – inferior articulating facet; E – spinous process; F – intervertebral foramen

2. In the lumbar region the vertebral bodies become more oval in shape and much larger to allow for the greater weight that it supports. The spinous processes are larger and more horizontal. The spinal canal is also narrower.

3. The lumbar facet joints articulate with a similar arrangement to the facet joints of the thoracic vertebrae. The main difference is the facets have rotated so that they are facing one another side–by–side. In the thoracic region they face each other in the antero–posterior position.

4. Spondylolisthesis is slipping of the upper vertebra on the one below it and typically occurs at L4/L5 junction.

5. L5 is typically larger than L1 and has some features of the sacrum. Indeed at times there is sacralisation of L5.

6. If the bodies are asymmetrical then there will be unequal forces passing through each body, which may lead to osteoarthritis and osteophyte formation.

7. G – transverse process; H – lamina; I – vertebral arch; J – vertebral canal.

8. The intervertebral joints are secondary cartilaginous. The facet joints are of the synovial type.

9. The spinal cord terminates to form the cauda equina which is found at approximately L1 in the adult and L3 in a child. Below this the dural sac ends at S2 and the cord is anchored down to the sacrum by the filum terminale.

10. Symptoms of cauda equina syndrome include back pain radiating down both legs, with urine and faecal incontinence, perianal loss of sensation and loss of sexual function. These symptoms represent a surgical emergency.

11. In a disc herniation the nucleus pulposus herniates posterolaterally as the posterior longitudinal ligament usually prevents direct posterior herniation.

12. The anterior longitudinal ligament lies anterior to the vertebral bodies along the whole length of the spine. The posterior longitudinal ligament lies posterior the vertebral bodies within the spinal canal. The ligamentum flavum connects the lamina of each adjacent vertebra. The interspinous ligament lies between each adjacent spinous process and the supraspinous ligament ascends along the tips of the spinous processes.

13. The extradural space consists of fat and the venous vertebral plexus (of Batson), which is a valveless venous plexus that is in communication with the deep pelvic veins. This is the route for metastasis of a prostatic malignancy.

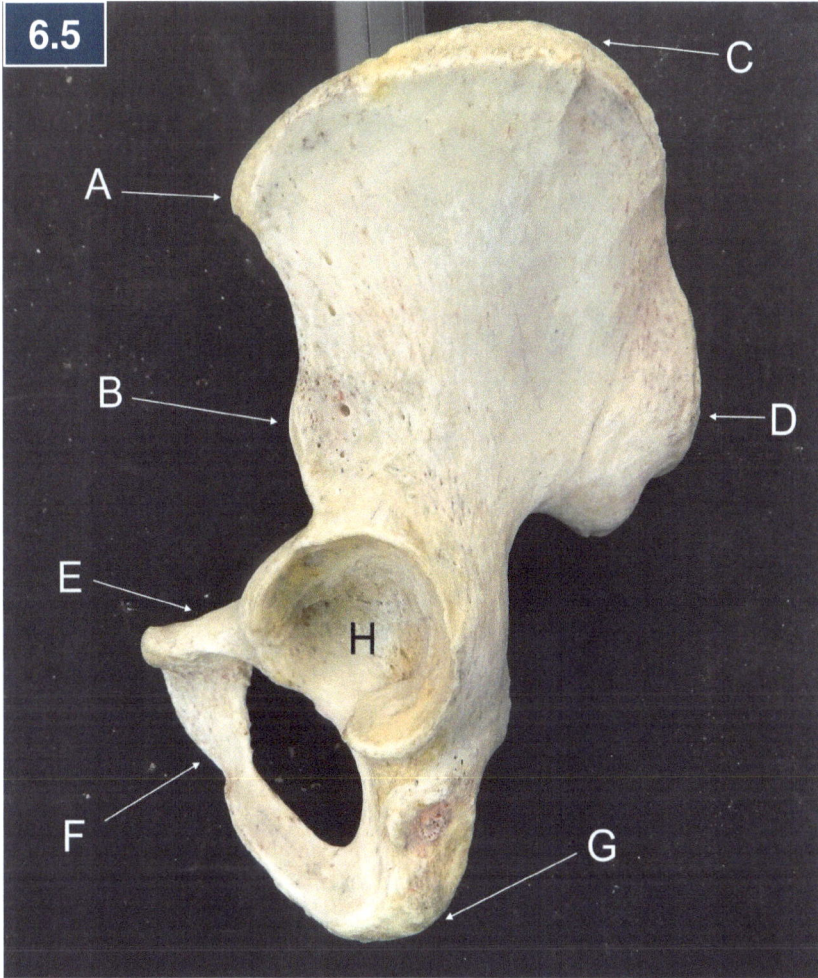

6.5

QUESTIONS

1. What is this bone, and which side is it from?

2. Name the three bones that it is made up of.

3. Identify A – H.

4. What muscle originates at B, and what is its action?

5. What muscles originate at G, and what are their actions?

6. What is the innervation of the muscles identified in questions 4 and 5?

7. What bone articulates with H?

8. What are three ligaments that attach this bone to H?

SPINE

ANSWERS

1. The left pelvic bone (also called the innominate bone)

2. Ilium, ischium and pubis.

3. A – anterior superior iliac spine; B – anterior inferior iliac spine; C – iliac crest; D – posterior superior iliac spine; E – superior pubic ramus; F – inferior pubic ramus; G – ischial tuberosity; H – acetabulum.

4. Rectus femoris, this forms part of the quadriceps muscle group and is the only muscle in that group to cross both the hip and the knee. As such it flexes the hip and extends the knee.

5. The hamstrings group (with the exception of the short head of biceps femoris) originate from the ischial tuberosity. The origin of the short head of biceps is the lateral border of the linea aspera. The hamstring group extend the hip and flex the knee.

6. Rectus femoris is innervated by the femoral nerve (L2,3,4); the hamstrings are innervated by the sciatic nerve (L4,5, S1,2,3).

7. The head of the femur.

8. Iliofemoral, ischiofemoral and pubofemoral ligaments.

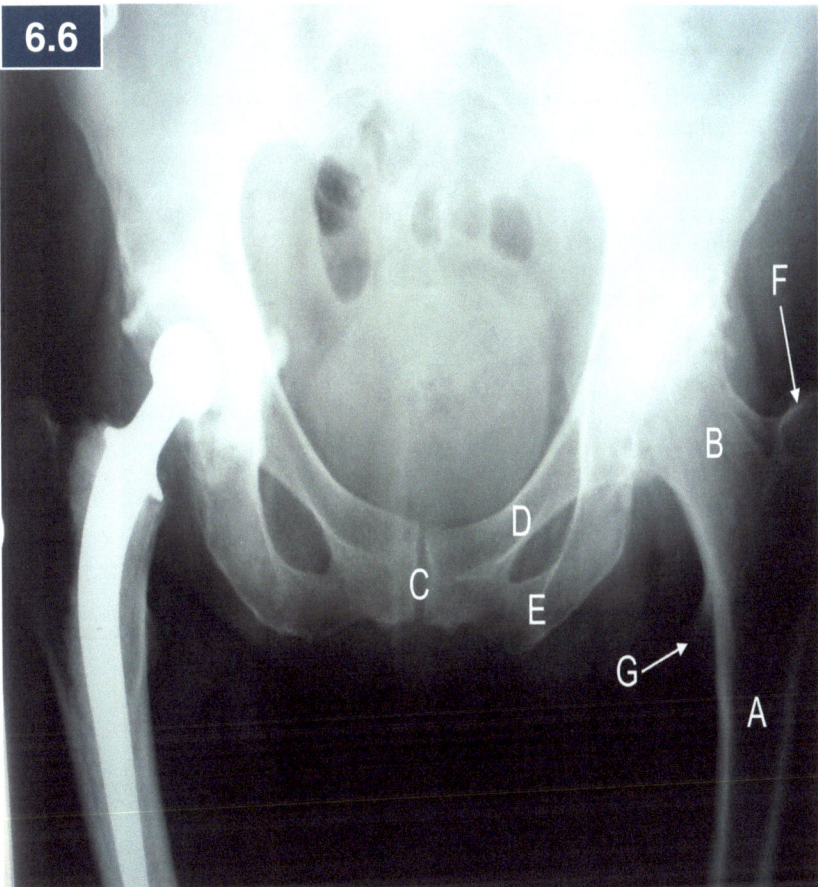

6.6

QUESTIONS

1. Identify structures A – G
2. What muscles attach to G?
3. What type of joint is C?
4. What implant is present in the image?
5. Describe the appearance of the left hip joint.
6. What are the classic features of osteoarthritis seen on a plain radiograph?
7. What surgical approaches do you know to the hip joint?

ANSWERS

1. A – left femoral shaft; B – left femoral neck; C – pubic symphysis;
D – superior pubic ramus; E – inferior pubic ramus; F – greater trochanter; G – lesser trochanter.

2. The psoas major muscle inserts onto the lesser trochanter. The ilacus muscle inserts onto a crest at the base of the lesser trochanter.

3. Secondary cartilaginous joint.

4. A right total hip replacement is seen.

5. There is evidence of joint space narrowing and periarticular osteophytes.

6. These include joint space loss, osteophyte formation, cysts and periarticular osteosclerosis.

7. There are multiple possible approaches to the hip joint, all with various advantages and disadvantages. These include:
   - Anterior approach
   - Anterolateral
   - Direct lateral
   - Posterior approach

6.7

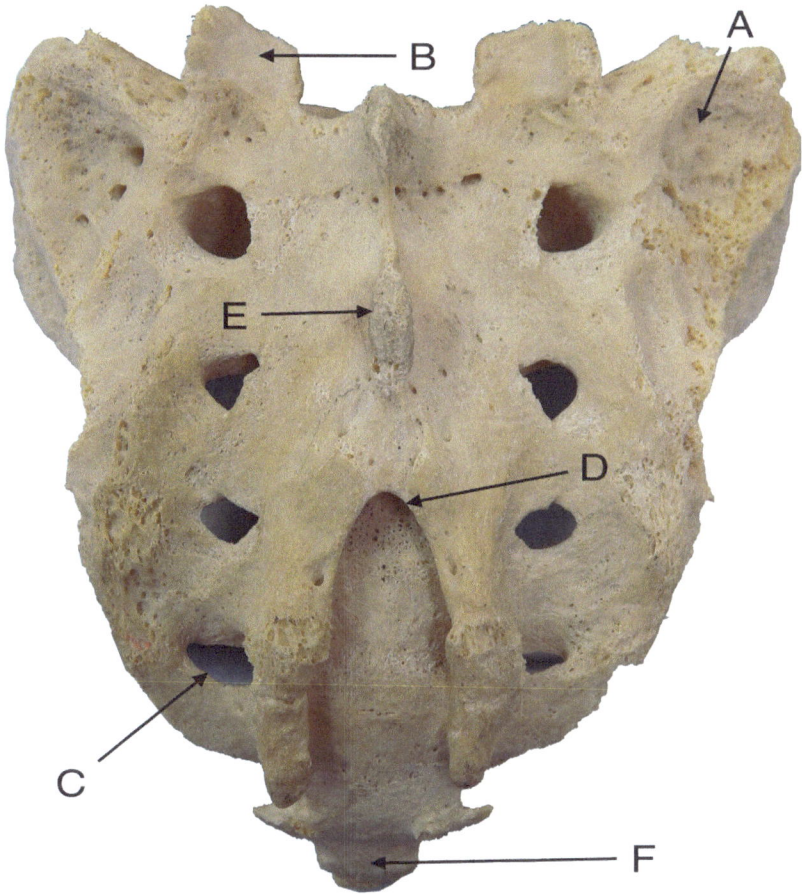

QUESTIONS

1. Identify A – F.

2. What articulates with the body of the first sacral vertebrae?

3. Which nerves pass through the posterior sacral foramina? Which structures are supplied by these nerves?

4. How can the sex of the patient be determined from the dry bone specimen?

5. Why may a needle be passed through the sacral hiatus?

SPINE

ANSWERS

1. A – ala; B – superior articular facet; C – posterior sacral foramen;
D – sacral hiatus; E – median sacral crest; F – coccyx.

2. The first sacral vertebra articulates with the body of vertebra L5. The body of vertebra L5 may be partially or completely fused with the body of S1, known as sacralisation of L5. Alternatively, the body of S1 may be completely separate from the rest of the sacrum, known as lumbarisation of S1.

3. The posterior branches of the sacral nerves pass through the posterior sacral foramina. These are mixed nerves and have visceral motor, somatic motor and sensory function to the skin and deep muscles of the back.

4. The sacrum is frequently used to determine the sex of a skeleton. The width of the body of S1 can be compared to the width of the sacral ala. In a male specimen the body of S1 will be notably wider than the ala. By comparison, in a female specimen the ala and sacral body will be of similar width.

5. A caudal epidural nerve block may be performed to provide analgesia or anaesthesia to the perineum and groin. The needle is passed through the posterior sacrococcygeal membrane that crosses the sacral hiatus.

SPINE

www.ingramcontent.com/pod-product-compliance
Lightning Source LLC
Chambersburg PA
CBHW041306210326
41598CB00011B/855